THE SCIENCE OF
NEAR-DEATH EXPERIENCES

THE SCIENCE OF
NEAR-DEATH EXPERIENCES

Edited by

JOHN C. HAGAN III, MD

UNIVERSITY OF MISSOURI PRESS
Columbia

University of Missouri Press, Columbia, Missouri 65211
Printed and bound in the United States of America
 First printing, 2017.
ISBN: 978-0-8262-2103-2
Library of Congress Control Number: 2016960888
∞™ This paper meets the requirements of the
American National Standard for Permanence of Paper
for Printed Library Materials, Z39.48, 1984.
Typefaces: Fontin, Caslon

Contents

Foreword

Raymond Moody, MD, PhD

PHYSICIANS AND OTHERS WHO TREAT terminally ill patients sometimes hear the poignant and heart-wrenching question: "*What is it like to die?*" Yet the answer always seems beyond the scope of the medical profession and perhaps even beyond the reach of human knowledge. This trailblazing book about near-death experiences provides a partial answer that informs clinicians and comforts dying patients.

Near-death experiences are fairly common among survivors of cardiac arrest and other severe medical conditions. Near-death experiences captured worldwide attention in 1976 and they have held the public's interest and stoked their imagination continually since then. These experiences are bound to become more common with the steady advance of techniques of cardiopulmonary resuscitation. Hence, this unique book is appearing at a particularly opportune time. Near-death experiences present truly interdisciplinary problems that concern clinical medicine, philosophy, religious studies, and the neurosciences in equal measure. Professionals in these fields will find plenty of clinically useful and thought-provoking information in this book.

The fascinating papers that this book brings together represent a variety of different perspectives. The medical physicians whose papers describe their own personal near-death experiences deserve our particular gratitude and respect. For their clear conviction that they experienced a transcendent state of conscious existence beyond the physical world awakens questions in clinical medicine about an afterlife. How should physicians and healthcare professionals respond to bright, articulate patients who report that they visited a light-filled after-death realm when they almost died? Clinical and philosophical issues are inextricably intertwined in this poignant question.

Clinically, the situation is usually straightforward. Physicians should listen thoughtfully to what their revived patients report. Then they should assure the patients that they are not alone in that such experiences occur frequently among individuals who recover after almost dying. Physicians should also acknowledge that such experiences often profoundly affect patients' subsequent spiritual lives. Interpreting such an experience should be left to the patient. In particular, attempting to explain near-death experiences neurophysiologically as hallucinations induced by oxygen deprivation to the brain typically alienates patients.

Besides, life after death is not yet a scientifically answerable, testable question. Rather, it is an important, traditional philosophical problem. And the old philosophical problem of an afterlife has intrusively manifested itself at the heart of clinical practice. Hence, it is not intellectually honest to avoid the question in one's personal reflections. After all, many brilliant, perceptive people of good judgment conclude from their personal near-death experiences that there is a life after death. How can the rational mind make sense of such an extraordinary state of affairs?

Modern medicine and the ancient discipline of philosophy may seem far apart. However, philosophical reasoning is exactly what is needed to grapple with the question of life after death. The greatest philosophical minds pointed out that those questions about an afterlife are incommensurable with the Aristotelian logic that underlies ordinary reasoning. Therefore, the emergence of the afterlife question within clinical practice of medicine presents exciting challenges calling for new methods of conceptual analysis. The time is right for innovative rational inquiry into the biggest question of human existence. This book, the first compiled by a respected, mainstream, peer-reviewed medical journal, is a bold step in that direction.

Acknowledgments

THIS BOOK IS BASED ON a series of editorials and articles appearing in ***Missouri Medicine: The Journal of the Missouri State Medical Association*** beginning September/October 2013 and concluding July/August 2015. Thanks go to our world-known near-death experiences scientific authors for their expertise and quality contributions. The articles are all reproduced by permission of the Missouri State Medical Association (MSMA), which holds their copyrights. No portion of this book may be reproduced without MSMA written permission. I wish to thank MSMA for the great honor of serving as Editor of *Missouri Medicine* since 2000. The production and design of *Missouri Medicine: The Journal of the Missouri State Medical Association* is entirely done by Managing Editor Lizabeth Fleenor. Without her skills, dedication, and expertise neither *Missouri Medicine* nor this book could be produced. MSMA would also like to thank University of Missouri Press for their expertise in the production and publication of this book and especially for embracing the importance of this subject and enthusiasm for bringing it to publication.

Finally, this book is dedicated to my intelligent, lovely and loving wife, Becky Hagan. Your life has meant everything to me.

About *Missouri Medicine*

The Journal of the Missouri State Medical Association

Missouri Medicine IS PEER-REVIEWED, AND content is linked with PubMed Central, which is the U.S. National Institutes digital archive of biomedical and life sciences journal literature. Content is indexed and can be found on MEDLINE, the National Library of Medicine, and EBSCO host databases. *Missouri Medicine* is owned by the Missouri State Medical Association and has been in publication since 1904. It has won numerous awards as best in state publication (Ranly Awards). *Missouri Medicine* also provides select featured content for www.medhelp.org the world's largest online health community which reaches more than 140 million users worldwide each year.

In recent years *Missouri Medicine* articles have been featured internationally: *Wall Street Journal; Outside Magazine; Runner's World; NBC News; General Surgery News; Anesthesia News* and major national newspapers. Besides having a national presence, *Missouri Medicine* is the largest circulation healthcare publication in Missouri, and its catchment area includes seven medical schools. Link to previous issues can be found at www.msma.org.

THE SCIENCE OF
NEAR-DEATH EXPERIENCES

The most important discoveries will provide answers to questions that we do not yet know how to ask and will concern objects we have not yet imagined.

John N. Bahcall, astrophysicist (1935–2005)

INTRODUCTION

The Science of Near-Death Experience

The Most Comprehensive Study in the World's Medical Peer-Reviewed Literature

John C. Hagan III, MD, FACS, FAAO

Physicians and all healthcare professionals must learn how to appropriately deal with patients who report an NDE. Let's get comfortable with near-death experiences.

WHAT HAPPENS TO CONSCIOUSNESS DURING the act of dying? Our best answer comes from people who "almost die" but return to life and recall events that occurred while resuscitation, emergency care, or surgery was performed to snatch life back from the jaws of death. As our medical and surgical skills increase, we can bring back patients who have traveled further on the path to death than at any other time in history. Their recollections often refute physicians' scientific explanation of how an oxygen-starved brain can produce such intense, vivid, and often corroborated veridical recollections. These events are now called "near-death experiences" (NDEs) and are often life-changing for those people who have them. The term NDE was coined by Raymond Moody, MD, PhD, in 1975 in his seminal book *Life After Life,* which is a perennial best-seller: over 13 million copies sold to date.

My own interest in NDEs began several years ago when at a party I asked a friend what he was reading. He replied, "*Evidence of the Afterlife: The Science of Near-Death Experiences* by Dr. Jeffrey Long." He added, "You should read it when I'm done. It's very thought-provoking. I think they are for real." After reading more than a dozen books on the subject, I concluded a multi-article peer-reviewed scientific study of NDEs by physicians and other scientists would be a tremendous precedent-setting achievement for medicine in general and *Missouri Medicine* in particular.

The *Missouri Medicine* near-death experience series republished in this book is the most encyclopedic and up-to-date in the world's medical literature. We used two criteria when recruiting authors: (1) esteemed physicians or evidence-based scientific researchers in the field of near-death experiences; (2) physicians who have themselves had a near-death experience. We preferred physician NDE accounts over non-physician NDE accounts because physicians are objective observers, they have direct understanding of possible physiological interpretations, and their scientific background lends added credibility to their reports.

Physicians and all healthcare professionals must learn how to appropriately deal with patients who report an NDE. Estimates on the number of people in the United States alone who have had an NDE vary from 9 to 20 million. As a group, physicians do not appreciate how often their patients experience NDEs or how to care for those who have one. This must change!

Many metaphysical questions are encountered in the study of NDEs. NDE reports challenge many of physicians' and scientists' deep-seated medical beliefs about what happens to brain function and consciousness at the threshold of death. NDEs make us scientists reflect, perhaps with considerable discomfort, on mankind's oldest and most profound questions: Where did we come from? Why are we here? What is life all about? What happens when we die? Of course questions and contemplation of death, the mystery of the terminal process of dying, and fears/faith/fatalism about the nature or existence of an afterlife are hardwired in our DNA from the onset of sentience.

In Chapter One, **Raymond A. Moody**, MD, PhD—the Father of NDEs and the author of books that have sold over 20 million copies—describes how historical records dating to ancient Greece contain descriptions congruous with the modern concept of an NDE. Moody's book *Life After Life* (1975, HarperOne) presented an initial collection of over 150 contemporary NDEs. The NDE typically includes many of the following: the mind leaving the body and traveling upward; passing from dark to a brilliant light often within a tunnel. The light, which is often interpreted to be God or the Supreme Being, is ineffable and transmits joy, peace, love, and comfort. Experiencers meet with deceased loved ones, friends, and relatives who welcome them. They have a life review in which they come to understand the meaning of their life and how they have lived it and how it affected others. They never wish to leave this unity with the light source of love. They return to mortal life reluctantly to help those needing them on Earth or sometimes involuntarily because they hear "your time has not yet come." Upon returning to their earthly body, most live a more purposeful, love-filled life. Thereafter the fear of death is generally absent.

Bruce Greyson, MD, Professor at the University of Virginia School of Medicine and a Co-Founder of the International Association for Near-Death Studies (IANDS), in Chapter Two reviews postulated scientific explanations of NDEs including, expectancy; birth memories; altered blood gasses; REM intrusion; toxic and/or metabolic hallucinations; neurochemistry; and neuroanatomy phenomena without finding a definitive explanation for NDEs. In addition to the positive aspects during and after an NDE, Greyson was the first to point out the occurrence of "distressing near-death experiences," which are disturbing, even terrifying, to those who experience them. He also noted that most people who have NDEs are mentally healthy and that one must not confuse or equate them with depersonalization, dissociation, post-traumatic stress disorder, or pathologic conditions such as Charles-Bonnet Syndrome.

Dean Radin, PhD, one of the foremost experts in using evidence and laboratory-based science to study NDEs, reports these conclusions in Chapter Three:

> With one exception, NDEs may be interpreted as unusual forms of hallucinations associated with the injured or dying brain. The exception involves perceptions described from vantage points outside the body that are later confirmed to be correct and could not have been inferred. Over a century of laboratory studies have investigated whether it is possible in principle for the mind to transcend the physical boundaries of the brain. The cumulative experimental database strongly indicates that it can. It is not clear that this finding implies the mind is separate from the brain but it does suggest that a comprehensive explanation for NDEs will require revisions to present scientific assumptions about the brain-mind relationship.

Pim van Lommel, MD, an eminent Dutch cardiologist has conducted prospective studies on patients having cardiac arrests during hospitalizations. In 18% of 344 successfully resuscitated patients they report typical NDEs. He also cites four other similarly designed prospective studies that found between

10% and 20% of 562 patients report an NDE. Van Lommel is the first in our series to raise the subject of non-local consciousness as a necessity to scientifically explain many of the presently puzzling phenomena of NDEs. Non-local consciousness is the thought-provoking subject of his book *Consciousness Beyond Life* (2001, HarperOne). His research appears in Chapter Four.

Jean Renee Hausheer, MD, is a respected ophthalmologist who previously taught at University of Missouri–Kansas City and now is Clinical Professor at the University of Oklahoma School of Medicine. In Chapter Five she describes for the first time her own NDE at Independence Regional Hospital (Missouri).

In Chapter Six **Tony Cicoria**, MD, Assistant Professor at SUNY Upstate School of Medicine, and **Jordan Cicoria** write about Tony's much publicized NDE that occurred in 1994 when he was struck by lightning. Post-NDE he had an obsession with learning to play the piano and write original music. He succeeded in both endeavors. See https://www.youtube.com/watch?v=tDtYkxSCV18. Both physicians describe their NDEs as positive, life-changing events that enriched their lives, reaffirmed their belief in God and removed any fear of death.

Jeffrey Long, MD, a Louisiana radiation oncologist, established the nonprofit Near Death Experience Research Foundation (NDERF) for collection, reporting, and study from NDE people worldwide. Please visit their website www.nderf.org to understand how universal and cross-cultural NDEs are. In Chapter Seven Dr. Long elaborates on nine lines of evidence that converge on the explanation that NDEs cannot be scientifically explained at this time. Among the most impressive of these nine are factual reports of events that have occurred in the past, or did happen in the future, or that transpired during the person's NDE that were physically remote and otherwise unknowable by the person. Other unaccountable events include totally blind individuals describing accurately vivid visual events during their resuscitations. Ninety-six percent of NDE-reporting patients to NDERF, many highly educated and scientifically trained, call their experience "definitely real."

Janice Miner Holden, EdD, Editor of the *Journal of Near-Death Studies*, a Past-President of IANDS, and a leading world expert on studying NDEs by apparently non-physical veridical perception (AVP), presents in Chapter Eight her research, and that of other leaders in the field on this fascinating subject. How can a person having an NDE experience during a cardiac arrest, upon resuscitation and recovery, report accurately events and occurrences local and remote in time and space unknowable even by a fully awake and alert person located in the same physical location as the apparently comatose and near-death person? AVPs represent one of the most difficult aspects of NDEs research that have yet to be explained by those scientists that ascribe NDEs to altered neurophysiology.

Penny Sartori, RN, PhD, is one of the world's foremost researchers in NDEs in children. In Chapter Nine she reviews her collective research, which includes NDEing children who later in life accurately describe events at their birth or infancy. She believes this shows that a mature functioning brain is not needed for an NDE. She argues against the brain being the seat of consciousness and that altered neurophysiology fails as an explanation for NDEs. She also notes children who have their NDEs timely validated have above average later life outcomes while those who do not have prompt validation have sub-normal life outcomes. She argues strongly for training healthcare personnel to recognize NDEs and quickly and properly validate them to those experiencing NDEs, especially children.

Nancy Evans Bush, MA, Previous President of IANDS, and **Bruce Greyson,** MD, recently retired Director of the Division of Perceptual Studies at the University of Virginia, in Chapter Ten skillfully present the little discussed "distressing near-death experiences" (DNDEs). Their review of over 30 years of NDEs literature concludes that DNDEs may occur as often as one in five cases and that both external and internal barriers to reporting them make them under-reported. The DNDE has distressing connotations to the hallmark events of the pleasurable NDE. The context of the DNDE is a "void" with feelings of aloneness, isolation, emptiness, even a sense of annihilation. Lastly, in the DNDE the "heavenly and redemptive" themes of most NDEs are replaced by a "hellish and damnation" experience. Much time and effort is required by these individuals to work through the debilitation and negative residua of the DNDEs. Three mechanisms often employed are "I needed that" in which the individual seeks to make amends in their life and become a better person. Movement to a dogmatic religious group is common. A second methodology is reductionism in which the DNDE is explained away or repudiated as a hallucination or an adverse drug reaction. A third group struggles for years trying to comprehend why the DNDE happened to them and why they cannot shake off its negative aftereffects. They often commit to long-term psychotherapy which is usually ineffective. Neither NDEs nor DNDEs are pre-conditioned by the conduct of an individual's life—a saintly person may still have a DNDE while felons and misanthropes may experience pleasant, redemption-giving NDEs.

Eben Alexander III, MD, former Harvard neurosurgeon, is the best-selling author of *Proof of Heaven: A Neurosurgeon's Journal into the Afterlife* (2012) and a comprehensive sequel, *The Map of Heaven: How Science, Religion and Ordinary People Are Proving the Afterlife* (2014, Simon & Schuster both). In Chapter Eleven he recounts his own miraculous full recovery from a virtually always fatal case of *E. Coli* meningoencephalitis and the complex NDE he experienced while in a septic coma. Drs. Radin, Van Lommel, Alexander, and pioneering neurosurgeon Wilder Penfield, MD, all deny that the complexity of the brain can account for the existence of consciousness. Alexander writes, "The truth is that the more we come to understand the physical workings of the brain, the more we realize it does not create consciousness at all. We are conscious in spite of our brain! The brain serves more as a reducing valve or filter, limiting pre-existing consciousness down to the trickle of the illusory 'here-now' in which we find ourselves in this physical realm." He continues, "The NDE community, as well as related spiritually transformative experiences of all stripes, provides compelling evidence that consciousness is fundamental in the universe."

In Chapter Twelve **Kevin Nelson**, MD, Professor of Neurology, University of Kentucky School of Medicine and author of several books, including *The Spiritual Doorway in the Brain* (Plume, 2012), provides what he feels is a "brain-based" explanation for near-death experiences emphasizing rapid eye movement intrusion and altered neurophysiology. He asserts that NDEs offer no insights into life after death or proof of what spiritualists call heaven. Whether you believe in some, all, or none of the interpretations and explanations of NDEs offered by other NDE authors as physicians and scientists believing in the scientific method, it is mandatory to read Nelson's theory of their causation.

In Chapter Thirteen, which concludes the book, **Eben Alexander III,** MD, examines in great detail the explanations of NDEs offered by Dr. Nelson in Chapter Twelve and finds them all wanting. He examines the writings of famous Canadian neurosurgeon Wilder Penfield, MD, and asserts that they are akin to his own and other NDE authors in the *Missouri Medicine* NDE series rather than the "physicalist" scientists that Nelson represents. Alexander also presents other esteemed world-famous neuroscientists who have left the physicalists' camp and no longer consider brain chemistry able to account for the existence of consciousness or the elements of thousands of NDEs that, studied carefully by science, defy scientific explanation.

As I have become more knowledgeable about and comfortable with NDEs, I have asked my patients who have had cardiac arrests or who were unconscious and almost died what it was like. Several have described typical NDEs without prompting. Physicians now seek me out to tell me of their own NDEs. It is a real clinical syndrome that physicians and health professionals need to recognize and be able to respond to appropriately.

Near-death experiences deserve greater unique and innovative scientific research. As Dr. Nelson presently believes, perhaps NDEs are explained by neurophysiology and are just brain "smoke and mirrors" trickery. Alternately, as Dr. Alexander and most of our other physician-scientist authors believe, we may be nearing the point where science proves that NDEs are real events occurring in a different, possibly spiritual rather than material, dimension and will ultimately be scientifically validated but are far beyond the powers of evidence-based science to understand and interpret.

CHAPTER ONE

Near-Death Experiences
An Essay in Medicine & Philosophy

Raymond A. Moody, MD, PhD

Near-death experiences are an ancient and very common phenomenon that spans from ancient philosophy, religion and healing to the most modern clinical practice of medicine.

Modern advances in medical knowledge make it possible to revive patients from increasingly severe, life-threatening injuries and illnesses, including cardiac arrest. Upon being revived, such patients often report experiencing life-changing alternate states of consciousness, which they tend to interpret in spiritual terms. Beginning in 1965, I interviewed several thousand individuals who had near-death experiences (NDEs) when they narrowly survived grave medical crises. I conducted the interviews first as a professor of philosophy and logic, then later as a medical doctor and psychiatrist. This paper is an overview of my research on near-death experiences, their historical significance, their characteristics, their sociological dimension, and their clinical implications.

HISTORY OF NEAR-DEATH EXPERIENCES

Near-death experiences are a perennially fascinating subject that bridges modern medical practice and ancient Greek philosophy. The Greek philosophers Heraclitus, Democritus, and Plato theorized about people known as "revenants" who had supposedly died and came back to life. Heraclitus mused, enigmatically, that the revenant is somehow appointed to watch over the living and the dead. Plato's most famous work, *The Republic*, culminates in the story of Er, a warrior who was apparently killed in battle. At his funeral, however, Er spontaneously revived and told a tale of moving away from his body and entering a complex afterlife world. Plato took stories like Er's seriously as offering some assurance of a life after death.

Democritus, the founder of atomic theory, was also interested in stories of people who had returned from the dead. In his writings, which now survive only in fragments, Democritus tried to explain "return from the dead stories" in terms of his favorite explanatory principles—atoms and the void. He noted that there is no such thing as a moment of death. In other words, Democritus held that the experiences of the dying result from the gradual winding down process of the body before death. Clearly people have known about near-death experiences for thousands of years. Such experiences must have been quite rare in antiquity and the medieval periods, since surviving an extreme injury or illness was much more uncommon. Scattered reports exist from those times, but the situation changed dramatically in the late twentieth century.

The last several decades of the twentieth century saw momentous breakthroughs in technology and procedures for cardiopulmonary resuscitation. Widespread use of these new techniques soon dramatically increased the number of people who survived a close brush with death.

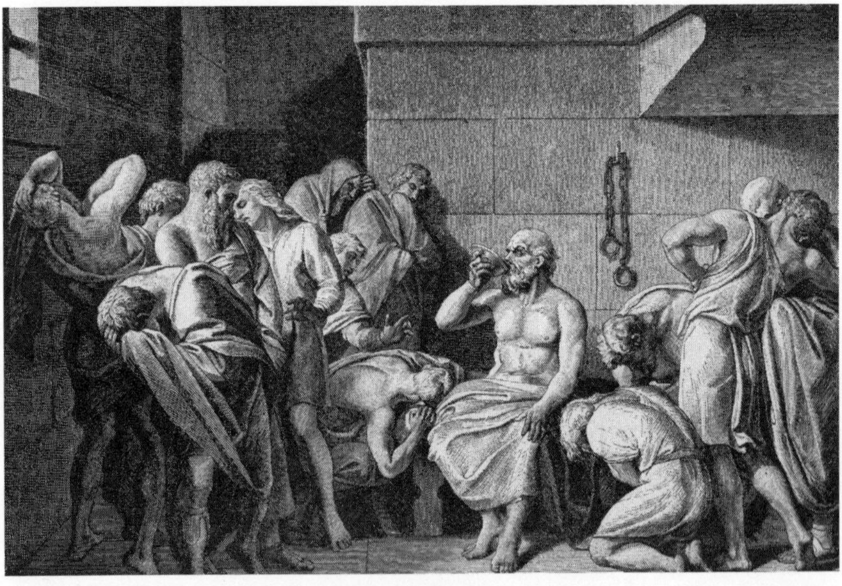

FIGURE 1 Socrates Drinking the Conium. Engraved by unknown engraver and published in *Pictorial History of the World's Great Nations*, United States, 1882.

By the mid-1970s, so many individuals had undergone near-death experiences that the phenomenon was bound to come to the attention of the public. My book *Life after Life* (1975),[1, 2] an analysis of about 150 cases of near-death experiences, was apparently the catalyst that woke the modern world up to this ancient phenomenon.

Since then, numerous physicians and psychologists have interviewed large numbers of patients who recounted near-death experiences. These physicians include, for example, cardiologist Michael Sabom, MD, psychiatrist Bruce Greyson, MD, cardiologist Pim Van Lommel, MD, resuscitation specialist Sam Parnia, MD, radiation oncologist Jeffrey Long, MD, psychologist Kenneth Ring, PhD, and others. All these authorities and others have published their findings and a large professional and popular literature on the subject has accumulated. A consensus has emerged among researchers that experiential reports of near-death experiences tend to conform to a discernible, common pattern.

CHARACTERISTICS OF NEAR-DEATH EXPERIENCES

Survivors of close calls with death usually recount their transcendent experiences in the form of a travel narrative. They tell us that their consciousness leaves their body and rises upward where they witness the resuscitation procedure going on below. They seem to pass through a dark enclosure toward a brilliant white light. However articulate they may be, they say that the experience is ineffable and indescribable; words are inadequate. They say that in the bright light they feel comfort, joy, peace, and love so intense as to be almost palpable. They say that they perceive the spirits of deceased loved ones, departed relatives, and friends who seem to be there to welcome them. These patients also say that they re-experience in vivid detail the events of their lives in a sort of holographic, full-color panorama. Although it takes only an instant, they report reviewing the actions of their lives empathically, from within the consciousness of others with whom they had interacted rather than from their original perspective.

Patients differ as to how they got back. For some, at one moment they were immersed in the light and the next moment they were back in their hospital beds with no sense of a transition. Other patients say that they were told, perhaps by one of their deceased loved ones, that they had to go back; that they had things left to complete. Yet other patients say they were given a choice. They could either stay in the light and continue that experience or return to the life they had been living. Most commonly, these patients say that for themselves they would have preferred to stay in the light; however, they chose to go back for someone else, usually to raise their young children.

Upon returning, these patients remark that their near-death experiences profoundly changed their lives. They say that their experiences convinced them personally that there is an afterlife so they no longer fear death. These patients say that whatever they might have been pursuing in their lives before—power, wealth, fame or something else—their experiences convinced them that the most important goal in life is to learn to love. Although they still find that goal as difficult to realize as anyone else, their near-death experiences commit them to pursuing love.

Not everyone who recovers from a near-death event reports a near-death experience. Nor does everyone who has a near-death experience report the whole, prototypical series of events. Some recall only a brief out-of-body experience with a view of their own physical body below, followed by a quick return. Others get only as far as the dark passageway, while others proceed all the way into the light. We do not know the reasons for all these variations. Notably, much of what "common sense" suggests about near-death experiences turns out not to be true.

First, NDEs do not seem to be dreams. Dreams seem less real than ordinary waking reality; NDEs seem hyper-real, that is "more real than ordinary waking reality." Patients describe their NDEs as almost the antithesis of dreams and deny dream-like qualities.

The occurrence of NDEs does not seem related to patients' prior religious training or beliefs. Many people with no prior interest or background in religion report powerful NDEs after surviving grave medical crises. NDEs are not related to specific medical conditions. Patients with infections, trauma, cardiac arrest, complications of childbirth, and many other diverse conditions have reported NDEs. There is wide variation in patient ages from the very young to the very old and every age between. Attempts to explain NDEs in physical or neuro-psychological terms have postulated complex seizures or brain anoxia. One problem with these explanations is that typical NDE phenomena often occur among deathbed bystanders. This is called a "shared death experience (SDE)." The bystanders are neither ill nor injured. NDEs and SDEs are not caused by brain hypoxia or atypical seizures.

SHARED DEATH EXPERIENCES

Bystanders or onlookers at the death of a patient may include physicians, nurses, other medical personnel, and relatives or friends of the dying. All of these types of bystanders report SDEs that are often indistinguishable from NDEs. For example bystanders sometimes say they saw a transparent replica of the dying person leave that person's body at the point of death. Or they describe leaving their own bodies and rising up to accompany their dying loved one part way toward the light. Onlookers at someone else's death also sometimes report that a brilliant light filled the room, they heard indescribably beautiful music and/or they perceived apparitions of the dead person's deceased loved ones. Occasionally, onlookers empathically report that they co-lived the "life review" of the deceased person. [See Editor's note, p. 17]

ORIGINS OF THE DESCRIPTION OF NEAR-DEATH EXPERIENCES

I first heard of a shared death experience from one of my professors of medicine in December 1972. Since then, I have heard thousands of such accounts from physicians, nurses, and kith and kin attendant at someone's death. I want to re-emphasize that all the same elements of near-death experiences reported by people who almost die are also reported by onlookers at the death of someone else. As incredible as this statement may seem, it is easily confirmable by any thorough investigator who will considerately and sympathetically inquire among people who were present at the death of others. I do not know exactly what the incidence or prevalence of shared death experiences might be but they are common and under-reported.

NEAR-DEATH EXPERIENCES AND MEDICAL SOCIOLOGY

In the late 1970s, dissemination of knowledge about near-death experiences, both in mass media and in the medical literature, caused a worldwide sensation. Books about NDEs sparked theological debates and speculation about the prospect of life after death. Popular movies and television talk shows enthusiastically took up the banner of near-death experiences. Almost forty years later, near-death experiences are still vigorously debated in every corner of the Earth. Numerous physicians have investigated the phenomenon and have been deeply impressed with patients' accounts of their near-death experiences. The topic remains a staple of television documentaries and newspaper and magazine articles.

This continuing fascination with near-death experiences has profound implications for the sociology of medicine. Advances in resuscitation techniques return to life a large number of people experiencing profound states of visionary consciousness at the very edge of absolute death. This is a prime example of how the progress of medicine can affect society in far-reaching and unanticipated ways.

Inevitably near-death experience reports have fueled debate on the possibility of life after death. There are no known rational or logical principles that allow reliable inferences about the prospect of an afterlife. Research into near-death experiences that is not rigorously rational may blur the line between medicine and religion. The best practice for physicians is to stick strictly to clinical and research concerns.

CLINICAL IMPLICATIONS OF NEAR-DEATH EXPERIENCES

What should a physician do when a patient recovers from an almost fatal illness or injury and reports a near-death experience? From talking with thousands of such patients, I find most simply want someone to listen to them noncommittally. They want to talk about what happened to them and to ventilate the powerful emotions and memories associated with their near-death experience. After listening, it also helps to reassure the patient that he or she is not alone, that millions of other individuals have had such experiences. Listening and reassuring them helps set them on a lifelong course of integrating what for most is their most profound transcendent event.

Intervening with their families can often save such patients considerable unnecessary discomfort and interpersonal conflicts. The family should know that the patient is not mentally ill nor are NDEs rare. Patients with near-death experiences are generally convinced from the outset that the experience was real and that they are not "crazy." They often worry that other people will make fun of them or doubt their sanity.

SUMMARY

Near-death experiences are an ancient and very common phenomenon that spans from ancient philosophy, religion, and healing[3] to the most modern clinical practice of medicine. Probably we are not much closer to an ultimate explanation of NDEs than were early thinkers like Plato and Democritus.[4] Puzzling cases of near-death experiences continue to come to light and the ancient debate about what they mean continues unabated.

[Editor's note: I have a friend of 40-plus years, highly intelligent, educated, non-religious, and absolutely truthful and trustworthy who volunteered having seen a "white mist" rise up from a dying great-grandmother's body and ascend to the corner of the room, linger, then disappear through the ceiling. My friend was age six at the time and had not previously shared this extremely common form of "shared death experience" with anyone.]

CHAPTER TWO

An Overview of Near-Death Experiences

Bruce Greyson, MD

An analysis of the incidence of NDEs among critically ill patients as documented in nine prospective studies in four countries yielded an average estimate of 17%.

NEAR-DEATH EXPERIENCES (NDES), PROFOUND EXPERIENCES reported by some people who survive close brushes with death, are important to clinicians because they often lead to pervasive changes in attitudes and behavior; because they may be confused with psychopathological states; and because they may enhance our understanding of consciousness. Proposed psychological and physiological explanations lack empirical support and fail to explain NDEs, which pose a challenge to current models of the mind-brain relationship.

INTRODUCTION

When some people come close to death, they go through a profound experience that may include a sense of leaving the body and entering some other realm or dimension, transcending the ordinary confines of time and space. Although these events had been identified as a discrete syndrome as early as 1892,[1] it was not until 1975 that Raymond Moody, MD, PhD, introduced the term *near-death experiences* (NDEs) for these phenomena. Moody described characteristic features commonly reported by survivors, including ineffability, overwhelming feelings of peace, seeing a tunnel, a sensation of being out of the body, meeting nonphysical beings including a "Being of Light," reviewing one's life, a border or point of no return, and coming back to life with marked changes in attitudes and with knowledge not acquired through normal perception.[2] A recent review of the accumulated findings from thirty years of research since Moody's seminal work has essentially confirmed his original description.[3]

An analysis of the incidence of NDEs among critically-ill patients as documented in nine prospective studies in four countries yielded an average estimate of 17%.[3] With advancements in medical resuscitation techniques, the frequency of NDEs has increased, and thus about nine million people in the United States alone have reported this kind of experience.[4] In the last 30 years, the near-death phenomenon has been investigated extensively.[5] Near-death experiences are important to physicians for three reasons. First, NDEs precipitate pervasive and durable changes in beliefs, attitudes, and values.[6] Secondly, they may be confused with psychopathological states, yet have profoundly different sequelae requiring different therapeutic approaches.[7] Third, clarification of their mechanisms may enhance our understanding of consciousness and its relation to brain function.[8]

One of the problems with research into NDEs is that, with a few notable exceptions, almost all NDE research has been retrospective, raising the question of the reliability of the experiencer's memories. Autobiographical memories are subject to distortion over years, and memories of unusual or traumatic events may be particularly unreliable as a result of emotional influences. However, memories of NDEs are experienced as "more real" than memories of other events,[9] and memories of NDEs have been shown to be unchanged over a period of 20 years.[10]

EXPLANATORY MODELS

Studies of near-death experiencers have shown them collectively to be psychologically healthy individuals who do not differ from comparison groups in age, gender, race, religion, religiosity, mental health, intelligence, neuroticism, extroversion, trait and state anxiety, or relevant Rorschach measures.[11]

Expectancy

A plausible hypothesis postulates that near-death experiences are products of the imagination, constructed from one's personal and cultural expectations, to protect oneself from facing the threat of death. Comparisons of NDE accounts from different cultures suggest that prior beliefs have some influence on the kind of experience a person will report following a close brush with death.

However, individuals often report experiences that conflict with their specific religious and personal expectations of death; people who had no prior knowledge about NDEs describe the same kinds of experiences as do people who are quite familiar with the phenomenon, and the knowledge individuals had about NDEs previously does not seem to influence the details of their own experiences; experiences that were reported before 1975, when Moody's first book coined the term NDE and made it a well-known phenomenon, do not differ from those that were reported since that date;[12] and young children, who are less likely to have developed expectations about death, report NDEs with features similar to those of adults.

Cross-cultural differences in NDE accounts suggest that it is not the core experience that differs but the ways in which people interpret what they have experienced in terms of the images, concepts, and symbols available to them.[13]

Birth Memories

Some authors have suggested that NDEs, with their dark tunnel, bright light, and going to another realm, could represent memories of one's birth. However, newborns lack the visual acuity, spatial stability of their visual images, mental alertness, and cortical coding capacity to register memories of the birth experience, and reports of out-of-body experiences (OBEs) and passing through a tunnel to another realm are equally common among persons born by Caesarean section and those born by normal vaginal delivery.[14]

Altered Blood Gases

A common assumption has been that anoxia or hypoxia, as a common final pathway to brain death, must be implicated in NDEs. However, NDEs may occur without anoxia or hypoxia, as in non-life-threatening illnesses and near-accidents, and hypoxia or anoxia generally produces idiosyncratic, frightening hallucinations, and leads to agitation and belligerence, quite unlike the peaceful NDE with consistent, universal features. Furthermore, studies of people near death have shown that those who have NDEs have oxygen levels the same as, or higher than, those who do not have NDEs.[15] Likewise, some authors have suggested that hypercarbia may contribute to

NDEs; but several studies have reported carbon dioxide levels to be normal or below normal during NDEs.[15]

REM Intrusion

NDEs have been associated with intrusion into waking consciousness of cognition typical of rapid eye movement (REM) sleep. However, the REM intrusion hypothesis is contradicted by the common occurrence of NDEs under conditions that inhibit REM, such as general anesthesia,[14] and by the finding of reduced REM in near-death experiencers.[16]

Toxic or Metabolic Hallucinations

NDEs have been dismissed as elaborate hallucinations produced either by medications given to dying patients or by metabolic disturbances or brain malfunctions as a person approaches death. However, many NDEs are recounted by individuals who had no metabolic or organic malfunctions that might have caused hallucinations, and patients who receive medications in fact report fewer NDEs than do patients who receive no medication.[14]

Furthermore, organic brain malfunctions generally produce clouded thinking, irritability, fear, belligerence, and idiosyncratic visions, quite unlike the exceptionally clear thinking, peacefulness, calm, and predictable content that typify the NDE. Visions in patients with delirium are generally of living persons, whereas those of patients with a clear sensorium as they approach death are almost invariably of deceased persons. Patients who are febrile or anoxic when near death report fewer NDEs and less elaborate experiences than do patients who remain drug-free and are neither febrile nor anoxic. That is, drug- or metabolically- induced delirium, rather than causing NDEs in fact inhibits them from occurring or from being recalled.[14]

Neurochemistry

NDEs have been speculatively attributed to a number of neurotransmitters in the brain, most frequently endorphins or other endogenous opioids, a putative ketamine-like endogenous neuroprotective agent acting on N-methyl-D-aspartate (NMDA) receptors, serotonin, adrenaline, vasopressin, and glutamate. These speculations are based on hypothetical endogenous chemicals or effects that have not been shown to exist, and are not supported by any empirical data.[17]

Neuroanatomy

NDEs have also been speculatively linked to a number of anatomic locations in the brain, including the frontal lobe attention area, the parietal lobe orientation area, the thalamus, the hypothalamus, the amygdala, the hippocampus, Reissner's fiber in the central canal of the spinal cord, and most often the right temporal lobe, based on purported similarity of NDEs to temporal lobe seizure phenomena. However, NDE-like phenomena are almost never seen in temporal lobe seizures, and electrical stimulation of the temporal lobes typically elicits fragmented bits of music, isolated and repetitive scenes that seemed familiar, hearing voices, experiencing fear or other negative emotions, or seeing bizarre, dream-like imagery, in addition to a wide range of somatic sensations that are never reported in NDEs.[17]

These putative neurological mechanisms, for which there is little if any empirical evidence, may suggest brain pathways through which NDEs are expressed or interpreted, but do not necessarily imply causal mechanisms.[17]

EFFECTS OF NEAR-DEATH EXPERIENCES

Positive Effects

Regardless of their cause, NDEs can permanently and dramatically alter the individual experiencer's attitudes, beliefs, and values. The literature on the aftereffects of NDEs has focused on the beneficial personal transformations that often follow. A recent review of research into the characteristic changes following NDEs found the most commonly reported to be loss of fear of death; strengthened belief in life after death; feeling specially favored by God; a new sense of purpose or mission; heightened self-esteem; increased compassion and love for others; lessened concern for material gain, recognition, or status; greater desire to serve others; increased ability to express feelings; greater appreciation of, and zest for, life; increased focus on the present; deeper religious faith or heightened spirituality; search for knowledge; and greater appreciation for nature.[6] These aftereffects have been corroborated by interviews with near-death experiencers' significant others and by long-term longitudinal studies.[17]

Negative Effects

Although NDErs sometimes feel distress if the NDE conflicts with their previously held beliefs and attitudes, the emphasis in the popular media on the positive benefits of NDEs inhibits those who are having problems from seeking help. Sometimes people who have had NDEs may doubt their sanity, yet they are often afraid of rejection or ridicule if they discuss this fear with friends or professionals. Sometimes NDErs do receive negative reactions from professionals when they describe their experiences, which discourages them even further from seeking help in understanding the experience.[18]

Family and friends may find it difficult to understand the NDEr's new beliefs and behavior, as many of their new attitudes and beliefs are so different from those around them. Difficulty reconciling the new attitudes and beliefs with the expectations of family and friends can interfere with maintaining old roles and lifestyle, which no longer have the same meaning. NDErs may find it impossible to communicate to others the meaning and impact of their NDE on their lives.[18]

Researchers have noted that the value incongruities between NDErs and their families lead to a relatively high divorce rate among NDErs. The effects of an NDE "may include long-term depression, broken relationships, disrupted career, feelings of severe alienation, an inability to function in the world, long years of struggling with the keen sense of altered reality."[19]

NEAR-DEATH EXPERIENCES & MENTAL HEALTH

Although retrospective studies of near-death experiencers have shown most of them to be psychologically healthy individuals, NDEs may be confused with several psychopathological conditions.

Depersonalization

NDEs have been described as a type of depersonalization, or feeling of strangeness or unreality, that mimics a state of death and serves as a sacrifice of a part of the self to avoid actual death. However, depersonalization would not account for the hyperalertness, enhanced affect, and mystical consciousness typically seen in NDEs; and depersonalization differs from NDEs in its age and gender distribution, unpleasant and dreamlike quality, and separation of the observing self from the functioning self.[7]

Dissociation

NDEs have been compared with dissociation, the separation of thoughts, feelings, or experiences from the normal stream of consciousness and memory that is an adaptive response to trauma common in otherwise normal people. Many NDEs share with dissociation the disconnection of perception, cognition, emotion, and identity from the mainstream of the individual's conscious awareness. NDErs may have a tendency to dissociate in response to catastrophic events, though not in response to everyday stressors. Symptoms of dissociation among near-death experiencers, though higher than among non-experiencers, are still within the range of the normal population and far below that seen in clinical dissociative disorders. The dissociative symptom profile of NDErs is suggestive of a normal psychophysiological response to stress, rather than a pathological type of dissociation or a manifestation of dissociative disorder.[7]

Posttraumatic Stress Disorder

NDEs may lead to symptoms of posttraumatic stress disorder (PTSD) such as recurrent, intrusive recollections of the event, recurrent distressing dreams of the event, diminished interest in previously important activities, estrangement from others, and a sense of foreshortened future. The incidence of PTSD symptoms among NDErs is higher than that among survivors of close brushes with death without NDEs, although it is within the normal range and far below that seen in clinical PTSD. The NDErs' profile of moderate elevation of intrusive thoughts, images, feelings, and dreams, but no elevation of avoidant psychic numbing, behavioral inhibition, or counterphobic activities, is typical of a nonspecific response to catastrophic stress rather than of PTSD.[7]

Other Pathological Conditions

In an autoscopy experience an individual perceives the surrounding environment from a different perspective, from a position outside of their own body. NDEs differ from autoscopy, seen in a variety of brain lesions, in that the observing self or point of perception in NDEs is experienced as outside the body, from which perspective the subject sees his or her own inactive physical body, rather than seeing an apparitional "double" (or more typically a portion of one) from the perspective of the physical body as in autoscopy. NDEs are more complex than the mental imagery induced by drugs, are more often endowed with personal meaning, and often occur in the absence of psychoactive substances. NDEs can be differentiated from brief psychotic disorders by their acute onset following a stressful precipitant, and by the experiencers' good premorbid functioning and positive exploratory attitude toward the experiences.[7]

NDEs in Psychiatric Patients

In a large sample of patients in a psychiatric outpatient clinic, among those patients who had come close to death, scores on every measure of psychological distress were lower for those who reported NDEs than for those who did not. The percent of patients in this study reporting near-death experiences was comparable to that found in the general population, suggesting that mental illness itself is not associated with near-death experiences, but in fact NDEs may mitigate the distress of mental illness.[20]

NEAR-DEATH EXPERIENCES & CONSCIOUSNESS

Some of the phenomenological features of NDEs are difficult to explain in terms of our current understanding of psychological or physiological processes. For example, experiencers sometimes report having viewed their bodies from a different point in space and are able to describe accurately what was going on around them while they were ostensibly unconscious,[21] or that they perceived corroborated events occurring at a distance outside the range of their sense organs, including blind individuals who describe accurate visual perceptions during their NDEs.[22]

Furthermore, some NDErs report having encountered deceased relatives and friends, and some child NDErs describe meeting persons whom they did not know at the time of the NDE but later identified as deceased relatives from family portraits they had never seen before. Other experiencers report having encountered a recently deceased person of whose death they had no knowledge, making expectation a highly implausible explanation.[23] These aspects of NDEs present us with data that are difficult to explain by current physiological or psychological models or by cultural or religious expectations.[22]

These features and the occurrence of heightened mental functioning when the brain is severely impaired, such as under general anesthesia and in cardiac arrest, challenge the common assumption in neuroscience that consciousness is solely the product of brain processes, or that the mind is merely the subjective concomitant of neurological events.[24]

CHAPTER THREE

Out of One's Mind or Beyond the Brain? The Challenge of Interpreting Near-Death Experiences

Dean Radin, PhD

Philosophers have vigorously debated the mind-brain relationship without resolution for thousands of years, so further discussion or reliance on anecdotes is not likely to resolve this question.

ABSTRACT

WITH ONE EXCEPTION, NEAR-DEATH EXPERIENCES (NDEs) may be interpreted as unusual forms of hallucinations associated with the injured or dying brain. The exception involves perceptions described from vantage points outside the body that are later confirmed to be correct and could not have been inferred. Over a century of laboratory studies have investigated whether it is possible in principle for the mind to transcend the physical boundaries of the brain. The cumulative experimental database strongly indicates that it can. It is not clear that this implies the mind is separate from the brain, but it does suggest that a comprehensive explanation for NDEs will require revisions to present scientific assumptions about the brain-mind relationship.

INTRODUCTION

Neuroscientist Francis Crick famously quipped that the mind—the self-aware, subjective aspect of the brain—is "nothing but a pack of neurons." Crick asserted that all mental activity, all of "your joys and your sorrows, your memories and your ambitions, your sense of identity and free will, are in fact no more than the behavior of a vast assembly of nerve cells and their associated molecules."[1] This proposal, which is now a central tenet in the neurosciences,[2] suggests that near-death experiences (NDEs) are best understood as hallucinations caused by distortions in neural activity as the brain shuts down. No other explanation is possible, because from the "pack of neurons" perspective mind and brain are identical, in which case visions of distant environments or discussions with disembodied entities are both examples of bizarre dreams.

Among counterarguments to such brain-based explanations is the observation that NDEs are reported even when the brain's electrical activity, as reflected in an electroencephalogram (EEG), has flat-lined.[3, 4] This would seem to rule out hallucinations and dreams because if the brain is completely inactive then the mind must also be inactive. So NDEs could not be reported, but *ipso facto* they are reported, and so mind and brain cannot be identical.

At face value this line of reasoning seems persuasive, but it has been challenged by the recent discovery that brains continue to show activity below what was once considered to be flat-lined conditions in deep coma and in the dying brain. In 2013, Kroeger et al. reported that a "novel brain phenomenon is observable in both humans and animals during coma that is deeper than the one reflected by the isoelectric EEG,"[5] and Borjigin et al. found evidence contrary to the assumption that the brain is hypoactive during cardiac arrest, and in particular that, "High-frequency neurophysiological activity in the near-death state exceeded levels found during the conscious waking state [demonstrating] that the mammalian brain can, albeit paradoxically, generate neural correlates of heightened conscious processing at near-death."[6]

Based on these discoveries, if NDEs exclusively consisted of dream-like images, however vivid, convincing, or unusual they may seem, then brain-oriented explanations would be plausible. But hallucinations do not cover the full phenomenology. Some NDEs also include perceptions reportedly from outside the body that could not have been inferred from information received through the ordinary senses, and that are verifiably correct.[7] This does not happen very often, but that it happens at all challenges the assumption that NDEs must be figments of the imagination, or that those reporting these experiences were discombobulated and, in a sense, going out of their minds.

From a conventional view "distant perception" experiences are often explained as coincidence, selective memory, confabulation, or they are simply ignored as impossible. But are such explanations correct? Is it possible to go out of one's brain without going out of one's mind? Philosophers have vigorously debated the mind-brain relationship without resolution for thousands of years, so further discussion or reliance on anecdotes is not likely to resolve this question. Fortunately, about a century ago a new approach was initiated in hopes of breaking the deadlock. Experiments were conducted under rigorously controlled conditions to see if distant perception was possible.

ORIGINS

In 1876, physicist Sir William Barrett from the Royal College of Science in Dublin, Ireland, presented experimental evidence in favor of what he called "thought transference" to the British Association for the Advancement of Science. Six years later, Barrett helped found the London-based Society for Psychical Research (SPR), the first scientific organization established for the study of exceptional mental capacities known today as psychic or "psi" phenomena.

Many prominent figures in science, scholarship, and politics became members of the SPR. The early roster included Sir Oliver Lodge, known for his contributions to the development of wireless telegraphy; Baron (John Strutt) Rayleigh, who was later awarded the Nobel Prize for his discovery of the inert gas argon; Rayleigh's spouse Evelyn Balfour, sister of Arthur James Balfour, Prime Minister of Britain; and Henry Sidgwick, Professor of Moral Philosophy at Cambridge University. American members included Samuel P. Langley, Director of the Smithsonian Institution; William James of Harvard University; Simon Newcomb; President of the American Association for the Advancement of Science; and Edward C. Pickering, Director of the Harvard Observatory.

Over the years, members of the SPR and other scientific organizations developed increasingly stringent methods to study reports of mind-to-mind communication, distance perception, apparitions, and related phenomena. Scientists and scholars of the day were intrigued, as we are today, by the frequency and the credibility of such reports, so they sought to establish whether reports of psi experiences were real or hallucinations.

Challenges associated with studying these mental phenomena led to a series of methodological advancements, some of which have become gold-standard tools in psychology, neuroscience, and medical research. They include the use of double-blind protocols to control for expectation effects, statistical techniques for evaluating human performance, the human electroencephalograph

(EEG), and methods for objectively consolidating and assessing replication rates across experiments, known today as meta-analysis.[8, 9]

Surveys of the general population collected by the SPR and others were used to classify and create taxonomies of reported psi experiences. Four categories proved to be most amenable to laboratory study. They were mind-to-mind communication (now called *telepathy*), perception of information beyond the reach of the ordinary senses (*clairvoyance*), perception through time (*precognition*), and direct mind-matter interactions (*psychokinesis*). Publications of experiments exploring these experiences attracted a great deal of critical attention, which led to new methods and designs to address potential artifacts. Improved studies were conducted, and this cycle was repeated over many decades.

EXPERIMENTS

The literature of psi research reports thousands of experiments and a growing number of meta-analyses.[9] It is not possible within the scope of a single article to do justice to this massive database, so one class of experiments will suffice: investigations of the claim of mind-to-mind communication, or telepathy.

Some may imagine that research on telepathy still involves the use of ESP (extrasensory perception) cards, which were popularized by Duke University psychologist Joseph B. Rhine starting in the 1930s.[10] Dozens of experiments conducted by Rhine and others were published, comprising a cumulative database of over four million card-guessing trials collected from the 1880s to the 1940s.[11] Analysis of that database persuaded many scientists that ESP was an established faculty of the mind. One example of a scientist who was impressed by the state of the evidence was Alan Turing, a seminal figure in the foundations of modern computer science and the mastermind who helped break the German Enigma cryptograph code during the Second World War.[12] In discussing the problem of how to differentiate between machine and human intelligence, Turing wrote:

> I assume that the reader is familiar with the idea of extrasensory perception, and the meaning of the four items of it, viz., telepathy, clairvoyance, precognition and psychokinesis. These disturbing phenomena seem to deny all our usual scientific ideas. How we should like to discredit them!

> Unfortunately the statistical evidence, at least for telepathy, is overwhelming. Many scientific theories seem to remain workable in practice, in spite of clashing with ESP; that in fact one can get along very nicely if one forgets about it. This is rather cold comfort, and one fears that *thinking* is just the kind of phenomenon where ESP may be especially relevant.[13]

Turing's opinion was prescient in that this line of research was indeed forgotten by most scientists and scholars. But it was also a victim of unfavorable timing. Rhine's work reached its pinnacle during a period in which it became fashionable for academic psychologists to deny the existence of any form of mental activity, including consciousness itself, largely due to the rising influence of psychologist B. F. Skinner's brand of behaviorism.[14] But psi research did not disappear entirely for a very simple reason—many people, including academics, continued to report psychic experiences.

By the 1970s, a new method for studying telepathy was designed to overcome two problems encountered in studies involving ESP cards. Those experiments were easy to conduct but the test design often involved guessing dozens to hundreds of cards in a row, so boredom and biases introduced by knowledge of previous guesses (the gambler's fallacy) were inevitable. These problems contributed to what came to be known as the "decline effect," a systematic decrease in performance over repeated testing.

The new design was called the *ganzfeld* telepathy experiment, where *ganzfeld* is a German word meaning "whole field." The technique involved mild, unpatterned visual and auditory stimulation. In preparation for a ganzfeld session, an experimenter E collected a large set of photographs (in some experiments video clips were used instead of photos). The photos were arranged into separate pools, each pool containing four photos as different from one other in content and appearance as possible. Later, when a test session began, E escorted the "receiver" R into an electromagnetically shielded room and asked R to relax in a comfortable, reclining chair. E placed halved ping-pong balls over R's eyes and headphones playing white noise over R's ears. Then E directed a red light to shine on R's face, and R was asked to keep his or her eyes open and to speak aloud any impressions that came to mind. E left the room and within a few minutes the ganzfeld stimulation reliably produced a hypnagogic, dream-like state in R. E continued to monitor R's shielded room to ensure that no ordinary form of communication could reach R.

Meanwhile, an assistant A escorted a "sender" S to a distant location where A randomly selected one pool of four images from the larger set of prepared pools, and then randomly selected one of the four images out of the pool. That image, called the *target*, was to be mentally sent by S to R. In some versions of this experiment, R's voice was audio recorded and transmitted by one-way audio link to S. This provided S with performance feedback to help optimize the sending process.

After the sending period ended, E—who, like R, was blind to the target—took R out of the ganzfeld condition and together they reviewed R's mental impressions while examining four images, the target along with three decoys (the three unselected images from the randomly chosen pool). The images they examined were duplicates of the photos handled by S (in more recent times they could be images on a computer screen), preventing clues about the target from accidentally being conveyed from S to R or E. After examining the four images, R ranked them according to how well each matched his or her impressions of the target during the sending period. If R ranked the target image as 1, the best possible match, then the test session was considered a hit. Otherwise it was a miss.

This method unambiguously established chance expectation, because if telepathy did not exist then the best that R could do, on average, would be to rank the correct target first one in four times, for a 25% chance expected hit rate. A ganzfeld test session consisted of a single "guess" in which R was free to describe virtually anything that came to mind. This obviated problems of boredom and guessing strategies that plagued tests using ESP cards, but it also required far more effort to gain a single datapoint. On average, the advantages outweighed the disadvantages, and today this simple design has been repeatedly tested in many variations for more than 40 years. Researchers familiar with these studies, including confirmed skeptics, agree that when properly conducted this method contains no known flaws that might produce spurious results.[15]

From 1974 through 2004, 88 ganzfeld experiments were reported. Together they resulted in 1,008 hits in 3,145 sessions, for a combined average hit rate of 32% as compared to the chance-expected 25%.[16] This hit rate is associated with odds against chance of 29 million trillion to 1. Arguments that this result might have been due to successful studies being reported more often than unsuccessful studies, known as the "file-drawer effect," have been analyzed and reanalyzed and critics familiar with this literature have agreed that selective reporting practices are insufficient to nullify the positive results.[8]

When the ganzfeld telepathy database is updated with new publications reported through 2010, 1,323 hits are reported in 4,196 trials, for average hit rate of 31.5%.[17] The additional data increases the overall odds against chance to 13 billion trillion to 1. These analyses have been published and critiqued in peer-reviewed journals, and similar successful results have been reported by researchers who explicitly stated that they did not believe in the existence of psychic abilities.[18, 16, 17, 19]

If scientific evidence were analogous to forensic evidence presented in a courtroom, then one could justifiably say that this one class of experiments demonstrates the existence of telepathy beyond a reasonable doubt. When conceptually similar experiments are added to the evidential database, including controlled laboratory tests of the "feeling of being stared at,"[20] and correlation of EEG[21-25] and functional MRIs between isolated couples,[26-28] the weight of the cumulative evidence is even stronger.

The bottom line is that there is now strong evidence, confirmed using Bayesian statistical methods that take into account analysts' prior expectations,[19] indicating that the mind can indeed transcend the physical constraints of the brain. This conclusion is bolstered by other classes of experiments that also provide strong statistical evidence for clairvoyance,[22, 29] precognition,[30, 31] and mind-matter interactions.[32, 33]

DISCUSSION

A century of scientific studies indicate that perception is not bound by the limitations of the brain, at least not by any means that are presently understood. Theoretical explanations continue to lag behind the empirical data, but this is common in the history of science. For example, herbal preparations containing salicylates were used for thousands of years before Aspirin's mechanism of action was identified.[34] And even with robust effects that are easy to demonstrate, like magnetism, it took hundreds of years before useful explanatory theories were formed.[35] Thus, given that no one knows how consciousness can arise out of (presumably) unconscious matter, it is not surprising that science has to yet provide a satisfactory explanation for telepathy and other subtle psychic capacities.[36, 37]

Theoretical explanations aside, how does the existence of psi influence our understanding of NDEs? The main implication is that it reduces the likelihood that reports of distant perceptions can only be due to confabulation or coincidence. In any given anecdotal report it is not possible to know with certainty that the information was obtained psychically. But experimental data suggests that it could have been obtained that way.

Does distant perception imply that a disembodied consciousness literally leaves the body, or that NDEs provide evidence for the persistence of consciousness after bodily death? The evidence to date is insufficient to answer such questions because everything we know about psi comes from tests conducted with living persons. Studies involving mediumship, which investigate individuals who claim to be able to communicate with the deceased, have attempted to probe the boundaries between life and death, but of course all such experiments ultimately involve reports from living persons; purported participation by the deceased is inferred.[38, 39] To further complicate matters, there is both anecdotal and experimental evidence that non-ordinary states of consciousness (e.g., dreaming, meditating, under the influence of psychedelic compounds) are more conducive to psi phenomena.[17] Given that near-death is a prime exemplar of a non-ordinary state it may be that some of the strikingly vivid aspects of NDEs arise because of clearer forms of psi perception that are filtered out by a normally functioning brain.

CONCLUSION

The bottom line is that NDEs in light of psi research suggest that one or more of today's assumptions about the mind-brain relationship are probably wrong. An improved understanding of NDEs may well be found to involve a host of mundane brain-oriented effects, but it may also include glimpses of realities that are presently beyond our imagination. Given the revolutionary changes in our understanding of the physical world over the last century through the development of relativity and quantum mechanics, it is virtually certain that the scientific worldview of the next century will include entirely new ways of thinking about space, time, and—given the challenge of NDEs—consciousness.

CHAPTER FOUR

Dutch Prospective Research on Near-Death Experiences during Cardiac Arrest

Pim van Lommel, MD

One cannot avoid the conclusion that endless or non-local consciousness has always existed and will always exist independently from the body, because there is no beginning nor will there ever be an end to our consciousness.

ABSTRACT

IN DUTCH PROSPECTIVE STUDIES ON near-death experiences (NDEs) in survivors of cardiac arrest, 18% of the 344 included patients reported such an experience of enhanced consciousness during the period of unconsciousness, during clinical death, during a transient functional loss of the cortex and the brainstem. An NDE seems to be an authentic experience which cannot be simply reduced to oxygen deficiency, imagination, fear of death, hallucination, psychosis, or the use of drugs, and people appear to be permanently changed by an NDE during a cardiac arrest of only several minutes duration.

INTRODUCTION

A near-death experience (NDE) can be defined as the reported memory of a range of impressions during a special state of consciousness, including a number of unique elements such as an out-of-body experience, pleasant feelings, seeing a tunnel, a light, deceased relatives, or a life review, and a conscious return into the body. Many circumstances are described during which NDEs are reported such as cardiac arrest (clinical death), shock after loss of blood (childbirth), coma caused by traumatic brain injury or stroke, near-drowning (children) or asphyxia; also in serious diseases not immediately life-threatening, during isolation, depression, or meditation, or without any obvious reason.

Similar experiences to near-death ones can occur during the terminal phase of illness and are called "deathbed visions" or "end-of-life experiences."

So-called "fear-death" experiences are mainly reported after situations in which death seemed unavoidable like serious traffic or mountaineering accidents, and "shared-death" experiences are reported by bystanders at the moment of death of a close relative. The NDE is usually transformational, causing enhanced intuitive sensitivity, profound changes of life-insight, and the loss of fear of death. The content of an NDE and the effects on patients seem similar worldwide, across all cultures and all times. However, the subjective nature and absence of a frame of reference for this ineffable experience lead to individual, cultural, and religious factors determining the vocabulary used to describe and interpret this experience.[1] Near-death experiences occur with increasing frequency because of improved survival rates resulting from modern techniques of resuscitation and from new therapies for patients with cerebral trauma. According to a recent random poll in the U.S. and in Germany, about four percent of the total population in the western world have experienced an NDE.[2,3] Thus, about nine million people in the U.S., about two million people in the United Kingdom, and about 20 million people in Europe should have had this extraordinary conscious experience. An NDE seems to be a relatively regularly occurring and, to many physicians, inexplicable phenomenon, an often ignored result of survival in a critical medical situation. After all, according to current medical knowledge it is impossible to experience consciousness during cardiac arrest or deep coma.

Until quite recently there was no prospective and scientifically designed study to explain the cause and content of an NDE, all studies had been retrospective and very selective with respect to patients. Based on these incomplete retrospective studies, some believed the experience could be caused by physiological changes in the brain as a result of lack of oxygen (cerebral anoxia), other theories encompass a psychological reaction to approaching death, hallucinations, dreams, side effect of drugs, or just false memories. Therefore, properly designed prospective studies in survivors of cardiac arrest were necessary in order to obtain more reliable data to corroborate or refute the existing theories on the cause and content of an NDE. We needed to know if there could be a physiological, pharmacological, psychological, or demographic explanation as to why people experience enhanced consciousness during a period of cardiac arrest.

THE DUTCH PROSPECTIVE STUDY ON NDE IN SURVIVORS OF CARDIAC ARREST

In 1988 a prospective study was initiated in the Netherlands.[4] At that point, no large-scale prospective study into NDEs had been undertaken anywhere in the world. Our study aimed to include all consecutive patients who had survived a cardiac arrest in one of the ten participating Dutch hospitals. This prospective study would only be carried out among patients with a proven life-threatening crisis. All of these patients would have died of cardiac arrest had they not been resuscitated within five to ten minutes. This kind of design also creates a control group of patients who have survived a cardiac arrest but who have no recollection of the period of unconsciousness. In a prospective study such patients are asked, within a few days of their resuscitation, whether they have any recollection of the period of their cardiac arrest, i.e., of the period of their unconsciousness. All patients' medical and other data are carefully recorded before, during, and after their resuscitation. We always collected a record of the electrocardiogram during the cardiac arrest of all patients included in our study. The advantage of this prospective study design was that all procedures were defined in advance and no selection bias could occur. Within four years, between 1988 and 1992, 344 successive patients who had undergone a total of 509 successful resuscitations were included in the study. All the patients in our study had been clinically dead and in the first stage of the process of dying. The Dutch study was published[4] in the *Lancet* in December 2001.

RESULTS OF THE DUTCH PROSPECTIVE STUDY

If patients reported memories from the period of unconsciousness, the experiences were scored according to a certain index, the WCEI, or "weighted core experience index."[5] The higher the number of elements reported, the higher the score and the deeper the NDE. We found that 282 patients (82%) had no recollection of the period of their unconsciousness, whereas 62 patients—18% of the 344 patients—reported an NDE. Of these 62 patients with memories, 21 patients (6%) had some recollection; having experienced only some elements, they had a superficial NDE with a low score. Because of the prospective design of the study, we also included these patients. And 42 patients (12%) reported a core experience: 18 patients had a moderately deep NDE; 17 patients reported a deep NDE; and six patients a very deep NDE.

The following elements were reported: half of the patients with an NDE were aware of being dead and had positive emotions; 30% had a tunnel experience, observed a celestial landscape, or met with deceased persons; approximately one-quarter had an out-of-body experience, communication with "the light" or perception of colors; 13% had a life review; and 8% experienced the presence of a border. All the familiar elements of an NDE were reported in our study, with the exception of a frightening or distressing NDE.

Were there any reasons why some people recollected the period of their unconsciousness when most did not?

In order to answer this question, we compared the recorded data of the 62 patients with an NDE to the data of the 282 patients without NDE. To our surprise we did not identify any significant differences in the duration of the cardiac arrest (2 minutes or 8 minutes), or differences in the duration of unconsciousness (5 minutes to three weeks in coma). So we failed to identify any differences between the patients with a very long or a very brief cardiac arrest. It also was established that medication played no role. A psychological cause such as the infrequently noted fear of death immediately before the arrest did not affect the occurrence of an NDE. Whether or not patients had heard or read anything about NDE in the past also made no difference. Any kind of religious belief, or indeed its absence in non-religious people or atheists, was irrelevant and the same was true for the level of education. Only the large-scale Dutch study allowed for statistical analysis of the factors that may determine whether or not an NDE occurs.

As a result of our study, we could exclude physiological, psychological, pharmacological, and demographic explanations for the occurrence of an NDE. We were particularly surprised to find no medical explanation for the occurrence of an NDE, because all the patients in our study had been clinically dead. Only a small percentage reported an enhanced consciousness with lucid thoughts, emotions, memories, and sometimes perception from a position outside and above their lifeless body while doctors and nursing staff were carrying out resuscitation. And because of some cases of veridical perception during resuscitation we reached the inevitable conclusion that patients experienced all the aforementioned NDE elements during the period of their cardiac arrest, during the total cessation of blood supply to the brain. Nevertheless, the question how this could be possible remained unanswered.

RESULTS OF THE DUTCH LONGITUDINAL STUDY

Our Dutch study was also the first to include a longitudinal component with interviews after two and eight years, using a standardized inventory featuring 34 life-change questions, which allowed us to compare the processes of transformation between people with and without NDE.[6] The question was whether the customary changes in attitude to life after an NDE were the result of surviving a cardiac arrest or whether these changes were caused by the experience of an NDE. This question had never before been subject to scientific and systematic research with prospective design. Among the 74 patients who consented to be interviewed after two years, 13 of the total of 34 factors listed in the questionnaire turned out to be significantly different for people with or without an NDE. The second interviews showed that in people with NDE in particular, fear of death had significantly decreased while belief in an afterlife had significantly increased. We were surprised to find that the processes of transformation that had begun in people with NDE after two years had clearly intensified after eight years. We saw in them a greater interest in spirituality and questions about the purpose of life, as well as a greater acceptance of, and love for, oneself and others. The conversations also revealed that people had acquired enhanced intuitive feelings after an NDE, along with a strong sense of connectedness with others and with nature. Or, as many of them put it, they had acquired "paranormal gifts." The sudden occurrence of this enhanced intuition, or non-local perception, can be quite problematic, as people suddenly have a very acute sense of others, which can be extremely intimidating.

The integration and acceptance of an NDE is a process that may take many years because of its far-reaching impact on people's pre-NDE understanding of life and value system. Finally, it is quite remarkable to see a cardiac arrest lasting just a few minutes give rise to such a lifelong process of transformation. For obvious reasons most people feel nostalgic about their NDE because of the unforgettable feelings of peace, acceptance, and love they encountered during the experience, and the feeling of being forced to return back into the body. We identified a distinct pattern of change in people with an NDE and revealed that integrating these changes into daily life is a long and arduous process because there is at first hardly any acceptance by oneself as well as by others, like doctors, nurses, family members, partners, and friends. This lack of acceptance can make the process of coming to terms with the experience difficult and painful. So the NDE is often a traumatic event with many years of strong feelings of depression, homesickness and loneliness.[6]

OTHER PROSPECTIVE STUDIES ON NDE IN SURVIVORS OF CARDIAC ARREST

Bruce Greyson, MD, who published a prospective study in 116 survivors of cardiac arrest in the USA,[7] found that 15.5% of the patients reported an NDE: of which 9.5% reported a core NDE and 6% a superficial NDE. He writes that "no one physiological or psychological model by itself could explain all the common features of an NDE. The paradoxical occurrence of a heightened, lucid awareness, and logical thought processes during a period of impaired cerebral perfusion raises particular perplexing questions for our current understanding of consciousness and its relation to brain function. A clear sensorium and complex perceptual processes during a period of apparent clinical death challenge the concept that consciousness is localized exclusively in the brain."

Sam Parnia, MD, and Peter Fenwick, MD, from the UK included in their prospective study 63 patients who survived their cardiac arrest.[8] They found that 11% reported an NDE: of which 6.3% reported a core NDE, and 4.8% a superficial NDE. They report that the NDE cases with veridical perceptions during cardiopulmonary resuscitation (CPR) suggest that the NDE occurs during the period of unconsciousness. This is a surprising conclusion, in their view, because "when the brain is so dysfunctional that the patient is deeply comatose, those cerebral structures, which underpin subjective experience and memory, must be severely impaired. Complex experiences as reported in the NDE should not arise or be retained in memory. Such patients would be expected to have no subjective experience, as was the case in the vast majority of patients who survive cardiac arrest, since all centers in the brain that are responsible for generating conscious experiences have stopped functioning as a result of the lack of oxygen." Over a period of four years Penny Sartori carried out an even smaller prospective study into NDE in 39 survivors of cardiac arrest in the UK.[9] She found that 23% reported an NDE: of which 18% reported a core NDE, and 5% a superficial NDE. She concludes that "according to mainstream science, it is quite impossible to find a scientific explanation for the NDE as long as we 'believe' that consciousness is only a side effect of a functioning brain." The fact that people report lucid experiences in their consciousness when brain activity has ceased is, in her view, "difficult to reconcile with current medical opinion."

SUMMARY SCIENTIFIC RESEARCH ON NEAR-DEATH EXPERIENCES

In four recently published prospective studies on NDE in survivors of cardiac arrest, with identical study design, between 10% and 20% of a total of 562 included patients reported an experience of enhanced consciousness during the period of apparent unconsciousness, during clinical death. With our current medical and scientific concepts it seems impossible to explain all aspects of the subjective experiences as reported by patients with an NDE during a transient functional loss of the cortex and the brainstem. Scientific studies into the phenomenon of NDE highlight the limitations of our current medical and neurophysiological ideas about the various aspects of human consciousness and the relationship between consciousness and memories on the one hand and the brain on the other. The prevailing paradigm holds that memories and consciousness are produced by large groups of neurons or neural networks. For want of evidence for the aforementioned explanations for the cause and content of an NDE the commonly accepted, but never proven, assumption that consciousness is localized in the brain should be questioned. After all, how can an extremely lucid consciousness be experienced outside the body at a time when the brain has a transient loss of all functions during a period of clinical death, even with a flat EEG?[10] Furthermore, even blind people have described veridical perceptions during out-of-body experiences at the time of their NDEs.[11]

NON-LOCAL CONSCIOUSNESS

It is a scientific challenge to discuss new hypotheses that could explain: the reported interconnectedness with the consciousness of other persons and of deceased relatives; the possibility of experiencing instantaneously and simultaneously (nonlocality) a review and a preview of someone's life in a dimension without our conventional body-linked concept of time and space, where all past, present, and future events exist and are available, and the possibility to have clear and enhanced consciousness with persistent and unaltered "Self"-identity, with memories, with cognition, with emotion, with the possibility of perception out and above the lifeless body, and even with the experience of the conscious return into the body. In my recent book[12] I describe a concept in which our endless consciousness with declarative memories finds its origin in, and is stored in a non-local realm as wave-fields of information, and the brain only serves as a relay station for parts of these wave-fields of consciousness to be received into or as our waking consciousness. The latter relates to our physical body. These informational fields of our non-local consciousness become available as our waking consciousness only through our functioning brain in the shape of measurable and changing electromagnetic fields. The function of the brain should thus be compared with a transceiver, a transmitter/receiver, or interface, exactly like the function of a computer. Different neuronal networks function as interface for different aspects of our consciousness, and the function of neuronal networks should be regarded as receivers and conveyors, not as retainers of consciousness and memories.

In this concept, consciousness is not rooted in the measurable domain of physics, our manifest world. This also means that the wave aspect of our indestructible consciousness in the non-local realm is inherently not measurable by physical means. However, the physical aspect of consciousness can be measured by means of neuroimaging techniques like EEG, fMRI, and PET-scan. There is a kind of biological basis of our waking consciousness, because during life our physical body functions as an interface or place of resonance. But there is no biological basis of our whole, endless, or enhanced consciousness because it is rooted in a non-local realm. Our non-local consciousness does not reside in our brain and is not limited to our brain, and our brain seems to have a facilitating, and not a producing function to experience consciousness. One cannot avoid the conclusion that endless or non-local consciousness has always existed and will always exist independently from the body, because there is no beginning nor will there ever be an end to our consciousness. For this reason we should seriously consider the possibility that death, like birth, can only be a transition to another state of consciousness. According to this idea death is only the end of our physical aspects, and during life our body functions as an interface or place of resonance for our non-local consciousness.

This view of a non-local consciousness also allows us to understand a wide variety of special states of consciousness,[13] not only near-death experiences, but also mystical and religious experiences, deathbed visions (end-of-life experiences), shared death experiences, peri-mortem and post-mortem experiences (after death communication, or non-local interconnectedness with the consciousness of deceased relatives), heightened intuitive feelings and prognostic dreams (non-local information exchange), remote viewing (non-local perception) and perhaps even the effect of consciousness on matter like in placebo-effect or neuroplasticity,[14, 15] where in EEG, fMRI and PET-scan studies functional and structural changes in the brain are demonstrated following changes in consciousness (non-local perturbation).

CONCLUSION

It often takes an NDE to get people to think about the possibility of experiencing consciousness independently of the body and to realize that presumably consciousness always has been and always will be, that everything and everybody is connected in higher levels of our consciousness, that all of our thoughts will exist forever, and that death as such does not exist. Only if we are willing and able to ask open questions and abandon preconceptions might research into NDEs help the scientific community to reconsider some unproven assumptions, not only about life and death, but above all about consciousness and its relation with brain function.

CHAPTER FIVE

My Unimaginable Journey
A Physician's Near-Death Experience

Jean Renee Hausheer, MD

> *I was forever changed by this experience. I was thrilled to have felt the wonder and beauty of the amazing love-light source that awaits us beyond the darkness here on earth. The transition and the Source are quite peaceful, natural, inviting, and comforting.*

DURING THE SUMMER OF 1977, at the age of 20, I experienced an extraordinary and transcendent event. I have come to understand that it is best described as an "near-death experience (NDE)." The insights of my brush with death altered my understanding of the meaning and purpose of life, forever extinguished my fear of death, and confirmed the ineffable wonder and joy of an afterlife. The series of articles on near-death experiences in *Missouri Medicine* address an important topic that has been sadly neglected in the medical literature and, for the most part, ignored by medical schools and the physicians they train. Accordingly I have chosen to go public and share my NDE with the *Missouri Medicine* readership.

THE EVENTS THAT LED TO MY NEAR-DEATH EXPERIENCE

My family and most of our friends love open water. Many glorious summers involved sun-drenched days and cool, starry nights at Lake Pomme de Terre. Activities included swimming, fishing, water-skiing, and racing over the glassine green water in our powerboats.

Summer was always a wonderful break from the rigor and stress of academics. In 1975, upon graduation from Truman High School, at the age of 17, I had entered the six-year program at the University of Missouri–Kansas

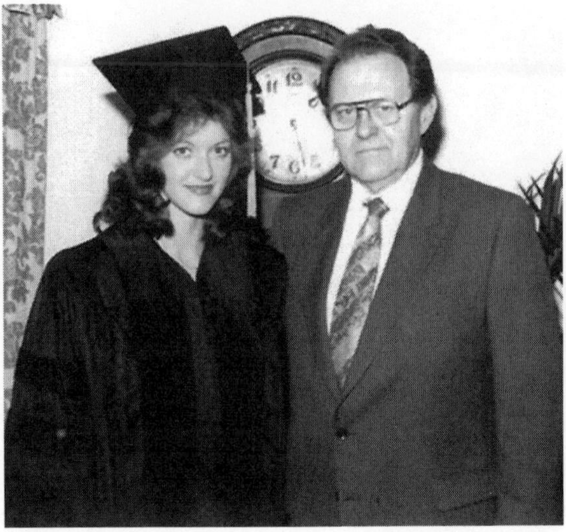

FIGURE 2 The author Jean Renee Hausheer, MD, and her father Herman J. Hausheer, MD, upon her graduation from University of Missouri–Kansas City School of Medicine in 1981. Dr. Hausheer's near-death experience occurred in 1977 while she was a medical student.

City (UMKC) School of Medicine. Academics were rigorous and physically demanding. We went to school eleven months per year for six consecutive years. Basic sciences dominated the first two years' curriculum. Clinical rotations started the third year. Although I was robust and vigorous, my parents carefully monitored my physical and emotional health, mindful of my young age and the stress that my studies and clinical work created.

Their concerns seemed justified in the summer of 1977 when, at the lake with my family, I developed what seemed to be a rather ordinary upper respiratory infection. My physician father (obstetrics-gynecology) had me rest and use a decongestant for my runny nose.

On a Saturday, two weeks after the onset of my "cold," I returned to UMKC to take an all-day standardized multiple-choice exam. Our entire class took these tests quarterly. In the first hour, unexpectedly and unexplainably, I developed very troubling intermittent double vision. With considerable difficulty, I completed the exam by shutting one eye then the other. By the time I completed the test, the diplopia was constant and bilateral ptosis was evolving. I called my father to report my difficulty. He was sufficiently alarmed to send me directly to an emergency room. Dad met me at the Independence Sanitarium

Hospital (now renamed Independence Regional Hospital). Meanwhile he arranged for a stat neurological consultation. My mother developed multiple sclerosis at the age of 36. My father and I both wondered if this could be the first manifestation of MS in me at age 20.

I drove to the hospital with one eye closed, where I was examined by a hastily assembled team of physicians. They decided to admit me. I was developing additional neurological deficits including severe bilateral upper-lid ptosis. This situation continued to progress over the next several days with a descending paralysis. My physicians narrowed the diagnosis to two possibilities: a Jacksonian variant of Guillain-Barre Syndrome or myasthenia gravis.

As the paralysis descended, I developed severe respiratory distress. Breathing became an exhaustive activity. Because of this dire situation I was sent to the pulmonary department for testing. The staff there performed a physostigmine challenge. Unfortunately, the amount of medication I received proved to be an overdose. Precipitously I was in iatrogenic acute respiratory failure.

MY NEAR-DEATH EXPERIENCE

I quickly slipped away as if in a dream. The last thing I heard was the therapist calling "code blue." Immediately prior to departing my body I recall telling her I just couldn't breathe anymore; it was just too hard and difficult.

I saw, as if from above and apart, emergency resuscitation efforts frantically start over my body lying on the floor. I viewed the frenetic activities around my dying body with detached interest. It was like watching a television show. My essence, my soul, my consciousness, my being, my spirit—whatever the non-corporeal quintessence of being should be called—was at peace and serene. Now I had no need for a physical body. Matter and gravity were no longer barriers to movement. Ahead emerged a wondrous, brilliant ball of the unimaginably whitest light from which emanated perfect love and peacefulness. Despite its infinite luminosity, the light was pleasing and caused my eyes no discomfort or photophobia.

As I departed, I failed at first to conceive that what lay below was my dying body. It was not a part of me and the surrounding medical drama was not my concern. It seemed natural to disregard and rapidly leave behind the limp human form.

This radiant ball of loving light initially appeared at a distance and rapidly surrounded my soul during my journey. The light sourced from a beautiful central ball-like brilliance that far exceeded that of diamonds. I became aware that this source of transcendent light was a peaceful, living, loving thing. From it originated the most tremendous transference of pure love and acceptance, far beyond human imagination. Very naturally and effortlessly, I was drawn to this living ball of loving light. As I moved toward the light the quicker it surrounded and insinuated itself within my soul. The love source and my soul merged within the light. We became one and the same.

Twice during this rapidly occurring experience, I realized my earthly body was dying and the loving light field was my soul's destination. Being only 20 years old, each time I thought about dying young, I could only think of one word: "No." As quickly as I would think this to myself, the movement to the light would halt like being suspended mid-thought. During each of these two "episodes of choice" there was a sharp contrast between this ball of living, loving light and the darkness from where I had come on Earth. The decision of whether to return to my life or move toward and into the light was a very difficult one for me. It fascinated me that I felt I was being offered a choice.

This living ball of light that emanated amazing amounts of the purest love totally surrounded me. Who I was and who this source of light was became one and the same. It was a welcoming home, as if the loving light source was now whole again, and so was I, analogous to merging two mists into one. The darkness from where I originated and its unpleasant feelings were completely gone. The second time I said, "No," I felt that I was being given a choice to proceed or return back to the darkness here on Earth. Once the process halted again, at the second decision point, a voice spoke to me. The voice wasn't male or female, was audible, and came from within this amazing living ball of lighted love. The voice surrounded me. The voice said directly to me, "Don't worry. It's not your time yet. Return!"

Faster than my journey to the ball of living, loving light, I suddenly awoke on a respirator in the intensive care unit at the Independence Hospital. I could see and hear all these people busy scurrying around trying to save me. I could hear them talking about how they noticed I was waking up. They were concerned that I would need emergency cardio-pulmonary resuscitation again. Of course I now had firsthand information; I knew I was going to survive.

The voice had powerful lasting meaning and finalized my continued earthly existence.

Once I got my hands on pen and paper, I wrote out a description to my father of my near-death experience. I told him that I knew I was going to be fine and my life was no longer in danger from this illness. I now knew my purpose here on Earth was yet to unfold. Now was not my time to die. My father observed how happy I looked. There was no wiping the smile off my face. I was at total peace.

I spent the next month in intensive care working hard to recover from this post-viral Jacksonian variant of Guillain-Barre syndrome. It took me a year to recover, including relearning how to walk and build strength and endurance back to normal levels. Over time my diplopia cleared. In spite of doubts about my ability to return to medical school, I was able to graduate with my class in spite of having missed many classes.

HOW THIS NEAR-DEATH EXPERIENCE HAS CHANGED MY LIFE

I was forever changed by this experience. I was thrilled to have felt the wonder and beauty of the amazing love-light source that awaits us beyond life here on Earth. I believe and choose to call this love-light source God. I will never again fear death for myself or others.

I've thought a lot, but talked little, about my NDE over the years. I share with you this conclusion. In the act of dying we are offered the opportunity of accepting and joining the ineffable light of pure and unconditional love. I've heard people concerned about the death of loved ones who didn't have a relationship with God. They fear their loved one traveled to eternal darkness. Because of what I experienced, my view differs on this topic. At the time of transition from "here to there," I was allowed to choose to be one with this peaceful loving ball of amazing light. At the time, I was a Christian and had a building and growing relationship with God but was still a greenhorn novice by all means.

October 10, 1993, I was privileged to suddenly and unexpectedly be at the bedside of my dying father, as he experienced an evolving myocardial infarction and severe cardiogenic shock. His face indicated immense pain and fear (probably worried about leaving our mom more than anything else). He was fighting for his life. I told him I loved him and would always take care of Mom for him. I said I would miss him very much. While his ailing heart was still beating, his face changed to an expression of total peace and comfort. That's when I knew his essence had transitioned away from his body. I looked upward, waved good-by, blew a kiss and told him again I loved him. The medical staff took his "living"body with a beating heart to the cardiac catheterization lab where they later pronounced him dead. I knew differently. I sensed and knew exactly when his spirit left his body.

I have been with a number of other family members and patients at the time of their deaths. I have seen their faces suddenly become peaceful with all pain and anguish gone. I know what they are experiencing. I know fully where they are traveling. I've been inclined to look up and wave goodbye to them. I am certain they'll choose to be one with the peaceful loving ball of light.

THE UNFOLDING OF MY PURPOSE IN LIFE

I am profoundly grateful I was given an opportunity to return to this earthly existence. My life is full and rich with many blessings. I went on to internship and ophthalmology residency at the Mayo Graduate School of Medicine in Rochester, Minnesota. I returned to Kansas City where I practiced from 1986 through 2011. I'm a healthy, happy 57-year-old practicing ophthalmologist. I have two amazing children and four stepchildren, each happily married to wonderful people. My husband Jim Meyer and I are blessed as grandparents of five grandsons and one granddaughter. My near-death experience allowed me to feel, see, and experience the profound joy when our soul post-death becomes one with the source of all love, peace, and light.

It is indeed an amazing journey to restoration with God the Father, who is the source of all light, love, and peace. Walls and ceilings have no boundaries to us beyond Earth. Our bodies are not necessary beyond Earth and are irrelevant after death. Our spiritual essence while here on Earth is what really matters. Nevertheless, we should take good care of our assigned bodies in our earthly journey. As physicians we serve in a noble profession working to maintain or restore physical and mental health to our patients.

I look forward to again meeting God the Father and my earthly father someday. What a wonderful reunion this will be.

CHAPTER SIX

My Near-Death Experience
A Call from God

Tony Cicoria, MD *& Jordan Cicoria*

The gift of life is greater than the sum of its parts and, whatever consciousness is, survives death.

IT WAS A BEAUTIFUL AUGUST day at Sleepy Hollow Lake in Athens, New York, in 1994. The occasion was my in-laws celebrating their annual group birthday gathering. About twenty relatives and their siblings were in attendance. While the children ran amok screaming and playing, I prepared the party barbeque. We had gathered on the second floor of a lakeside pavilion. The ground level included picnic tables and barbeque pits. A payphone was attached to the wall on the side of the building.

As the thought occurred to me to call my mother and check on her, I remember seeing a few light sprinkles of rain. In the midst of the revelry and chaos, and unbeknownst to me, the beautiful sunny day had surrendered to powerful dark storm clouds moving swiftly in over the lake. I ambled around the building to the pay phone and dialed my mother's familiar number. I let the phone ring eight times, but there was no answer. With my left hand I pulled the phone hand piece away from my face to hang it up. When it was about a foot away from my face, I heard a deafening crack. Simultaneously I saw a brilliant flash of light exit the phone hand piece I was holding. A powerful bolt of lightning had struck the pavilion, traversed through the phone striking me in the face, as its massive electrical charge raced to ground.

MY NEAR-DEATH EXPERIENCE

The force of the lightning blast threw my body backwards like a rag doll. Despite the stunning physical trauma, I realized something strange and inexplicable was happening. As my body was blown backwards, I felt "me" move forward instead. Yet I seemed also to stand motionless and bewildered staring at the phone dangling in front of me. Nothing made sense.

At that moment, I heard my mother-in-law scream from the top of the stairs above me. She raced down the stairs toward me. I felt like a deer in the headlights. As she approached I could see she was looking beyond me to my right and headed in that direction. She was oblivious to me standing there. I turned to see where she was going. Suddenly, I realized what was going on. A motionless body was lying on the ground some ten feet behind me. To appearances the person was dead. To inspection the person resembled me. To my astonishment another look confirmed it was me!

I watched as a woman who had been waiting to use the phone dropped to her knees and began CPR. I spoke to the people around my body but they could not see or hear me; I could see and hear everything they did and said. It suddenly occurred to me that I was thinking normal thoughts, in the same mental vernacular I had always possessed. At that moment I suddenly had one simple, ineloquent and rude thought, "Holy shit, I'm dead."

This cosmic realization of consciousness meant that my self-awareness was no longer in the lifeless body on the ground. I, whatever I was now, was capable of thought and reason. Interestingly there was no strong emotion accompanying my apparent death. I was shocked, certainly, but otherwise I felt no reaction to what should have been the most emotional of life's events.

Seeing no point in staying with my body, my thoughts then moved to walking away. I turned and started to climb the stairs to where I knew my family still was. As I started to climb I looked down at the stairs like I would normally do. I saw that as I reached the third stair, my legs began to dissolve. I remember being disconcerted that, by the time I reached the top of the stairs, I had lost all form entirely and instead was just a ball of energy and thought. My mind was racing frantically trying to record and make sense of what was happening.

At the top of the first flight, the stairs went up and left into the second flight. Instead of bothering with the stairs, I passed through the wall into the room where everyone was. I went diagonally through the room, over my wife who was painting children's faces. She had one child in front of her, one behind that person and one to the left. I had a clear realization that my family would be fine. Dispassionately, I departed from the building.

Once outside the building, I was immersed in a bluish white light that had a shimmering appearance as if I were swimming underwater in a crystal clear stream. The sunlight was penetrating through it. The visual was accompanied by a feeling of absolute love and peace.

What does the term "absolute love and peace" mean? For example, scientists use the term "absolute zero" to describe a temperature at which no molecular motion exists; a singular and pure state. That was what I felt; I had fallen into a pure positive flow of energy. I could see the flow of this energy. I could see it flow through the fabric of everything. I reasoned that this energy was quantifiable. It was something measurable and palpable. As I flowed in the current of this stream, which seemed to have both velocity and direction, I saw some of the high points and low points in my life pass by, but nothing in depth. I became ecstatic at the possibility of where I was going. I was aware of every moment of this experience, conscious of every millisecond, even though I could feel that time did not exist. I remember thinking, "This is the greatest thing that can ever happen to anyone."

Suddenly, I was back in my body. It was so painful. My mouth burned and my left foot felt like someone had stuck a red-hot poker through my ankle. I was still unconscious, but I could feel the woman who was doing CPR stop and kneel beside me. It seemed like minutes before I could open my eyes. I wanted to say to her, "Thank you for helping me." Nonsensically, all that came out was, "It's okay, I'm a doctor."

Shortly after I regained consciousness, camp security arrived and requested that an ambulance be called, which, to their frustration, I promptly refused. Although I realized I probably made little sense, the truth about lightning strikes is that you are either dead or alive, and there is not much in between. In retrospect it is obvious I wasn't thinking clearly, but at the time, I was still reeling from what I had just experienced. My family drove me the two and a half hours home to Oneonta, New York, wobbly and confused. Once there, I saw my local cardiologist and neurologist, who did all the appropriate tests and examinations. They told me how lucky I was to be alive.

I was able to resume work two weeks after the initial lightning strike when my brain seemed to function normally again. In the weeks and months after the lightning strike, however, I changed in many ways. The story of my developing musical ability and composition as a result of this event has been touched on in several books and documentaries.[1,2,3,4,5] (See facing page)

CAN SCIENCE EXPLAIN NDE/OBE?

I had experienced what Raymond Moody, MD, defined as a near-death experience.[6] For the purpose of this chapter, I am going to focus primarily on the experiential aspect of NDEs and attempt to apply scientific reasoning to what may defy explanation with our current knowledge.

As a physician and scientist, I think it is extremely important to attempt a logical explanation of what happened and to examine what I experienced that fateful day. As an individual, however, I also think it is extremely important to appreciate the indescribable miracle that I experienced. I was presumed dead on the ground, yet I was later able to see and verify things that had been happening around me and that happened in another room where it was physically impossible for me to have seen. Both are imperative variables in arriving at a viable conclusion to this enigmatic event.

My friend and colleague the eminent neurologist and renowned author Oliver Sacks, MD, assures me that I was hallucinating ... but was I? Dr. Sacks has described hallucinations associated with "ecstatic" seizures in temporal lobe epilepsy that certainly sound like some descriptions by people who have had actual NDEs.[7] However, numerous reports have been presented and verified in which NDE experiencers have been able to describe accurately and in incredible visual and auditory detail their NDEs. A case in point is that of Pam Reynolds, described in Michael Sabom, MD's book, *Light and Death*[8] and further studied by Holden[9] and Woerlee.[10] Reynolds was a patient who had an NDE during a neurosurgical procedure called "standstill" pioneered by Robert Spetzler, MD, at the Barrow Neurosurgical Institute. This procedure was used during Reynolds' brain aneurysm resection. She had an induced cardiac arrest and the brain was monitored and was documented to be isoelectric and nonreactive. Just before the standstill procedure was begun, Reynolds was deeply anesthetized, with her eyes taped shut and a sheet over her head. Her brain activity was monitored in more than one way to confirm that her anesthesia was complete and yet she described "popping" out of her body—having an NDE, whereupon she was able to describe sounds, "see" where people were

THE ELECTRIFYING STORY OF THE ACCIDENTAL PIANIST & COMPOSER

ABOUT TWO WEEKS AFTER BEING struck by lightning and my near-death experience, I began to have an insatiable desire to listen to classical piano music. This was a startling departure from previous musical interests. I was a child of the 1960s and was raised on rock and roll. Even as an adult I was only interested in classic rock. When I was seven, my mother insisted I take piano lessons for a year. Dutifully and reluctantly I did. I had no interest in the piano and would much rather fish or play sports. I abandoned the piano rather quickly. Now, dare I say like a bolt out of the blue, I was obsessed by the need to hear classical piano music.

I live in rural New York; I had to drive 60 minutes to Albany to even find CDs of classical piano. When I walked into the music store, a CD of Vladimir Ashkenazy playing his favorite Chopin seemed to fly into my hands. I listened repeatedly throughout the day. Within two weeks I realized I had to learn how to play the music on the CD. Unfortunately, I did not have a piano and remembered nothing from my childhood lessons. Several days after that realization, our babysitter asked if she could store her old piano with us for a year. Now that I had a piano, I promptly went to the music store and purchased some beginner's books on learning to play the piano. I also ordered all the sheet music listed on the CD that I listened to daily.

A few months after the piano came to live with us, I had a dream. This was not an ordinary dream, though—it was like an out-of-body experience. In the dream, I walked up behind myself and saw that I was sitting at the piano and was playing music in a concert hall. It was so real. I later drew a picture of the inside of the theater. I watched myself playing and suddenly realized that this was not someone else's music being played, it was my own. I listened to the music intently as it climaxed in a crescendo that woke me from a sound sleep. It was 3:15 A.M. I got up and went out to the piano to try to play some of what I heard despite having no idea how to write music, let alone play it. Frustrated, I went back to bed.

From that moment on, whenever I sat to play piano, the music would start to play in my head like a recording. If I tried to ignore it, it became more insistent. I became obsessed with the piano and came to believe the only reason I survived the lightning was because of the music. I practiced in the morning from 4:00 A.M. to 6:30 A.M. before work, worked 12 hours, gave our kids their baths and tucked them into bed with a goodnight song. Then I was back at the piano until my eyes could no longer focus. Every day I would write down a few notes or measures of my music and throw them in a drawer for later use. It was shortly thereafter that I became aware of my own ineptitude for self-teaching and began piano lessons with Sandra Campbell McKane, a Julliard graduate and professor of music at Hartwick College. The year was 1998.

I continued along this difficult path of piano competency. Annually, I spent a week at Sonata Piano Camp in Bennington, Vermont. In 2006, I met Erica Van der Linde Feidner who knew Oliver Sacks, MD. Erica knew he was writing a book on music and the brain. Through a complex sequence of events, Dr. Sacks interviewed me in August of 2006. At the end of that day, as we shook hands in his doorway, he looked into my eyes as if looking through me and said, "The music from the dream went through an awful lot of trouble to get here, the least you can do is write it." I was shaken by what he said; I went home and bought a Sibelius music writing program. I wrote bits and pieces of an original composition. I spent the next seven months writing frantically every day after work. Dr. Sack's book, *Musicophilia: Tales of Music and the Brain*, came out in 2007. I gave my first public concert in 2008 at the Goodyear Performing Arts Theater at State University College at Oneonta in New York. The music was recorded on CD and is available at CDBaby.com.

A YouTube video of me at the Mozart House in Vienna, Austria, playing "The Lightning Sonata," one of my original compositions, can be found at www.youtube.com/watch?v=tDtYkxSCV18.

---

standing, and describe the shape of surgical instruments used on her that she could not have seen physically. Dr. Gerald Woerlee[10] claims she may have had moments of light anesthesia, which certainly can happen in surgery, but that would allow only auditory, not visual recognition. She was able to mimic the sound of a brutish instrument called a Midas Rex that was used to cut through her skull. More importantly she was able to accurately describe what it looked like in lay terms.

An extensive number of cardiac arrest cases have been recorded with similar NDEs. Pim van Lommel, MD, a cardiologist in the Netherlands, did a prospective analysis of 509 successful resuscitations in 344 Dutch patients who suffered a cardiac arrest.[11,12,13] Of those, 18% had an NDE. In other studies, the percentage varies for adult cardiac arrest victims who recall an NDE.[14] Morse[15] found 85% in children. An obvious question is why not all? Ring[16] found that blind people who had experienced NDEs also reported veridical perception in which perceptions that were impossible to observe from the vantage point of their physical body, and sometimes that totally contradicted their expectations at the time, were later verified to be accurate.

WHAT DO THE SKEPTICS SAY?

Despite the strength of evidence in support of the reality of NDEs, many authorities still believe it is the work of a dying brain. Some of the controversy comes from studies that can simulate an experience that has some shared characteristics with actual NDEs. Those studies go back to Wilder Penfield's physical stimulation of the brain in patients.[17,18] Olaf Blanke, et al.[19] was able to recreate a partial out-of-body experience (OBE) in patients when electrodes were stimulated in the temporal lobe/amygdala region of the brain. Nelson et al.[20, 21] ascribes the arousal/REM system as an integral part in the expression of NDEs and that hypoxia and cerebral ischemia are influential in the expression of the NDEs. Some new studies in rats by Jimo Borjigin et al.[22] and Chawla et al.[23] in humans suggest that within 30 seconds after cardiac arrest there is a transient surge of synchronous high-frequency gamma oscillations (a neuronal feature thought to underpin consciousness in humans) that precedes isoelectric EEG (flat line) or brain death. These authors make a giant leap to suggest this mechanism underlies NDEs. That hypothesis would negate cases of documented cardiac arrest and brain death where patients have returned to life after death and brought back information they would have no possible way of obtaining through mediation of the senses and the brain.[24, 25]

OTHER THEORIES AND NOTIONS

The notion of consciousness surviving death is not new. Plato's story of Er in *The Republic*[26] and Pythagoras,[27] who believed God created souls as spirit entities whose goal is to merge with the divine . . . able to be eternal, transmigrate, and reincarnate, are but two examples. There are many books detailing the science of NDEs and a vast compendium of credible cases supporting the survival of consciousness.[28, 12] I think there is certainly something inherent in the temporal lobe/amygdala area that has a connection to what people experience as an NDE, an OBE, autoscopy (the experience in which an individual perceives the surrounding environment from a different perspective, from a position outside of his or her own body) or other unexplained phenomena.[29] There is experimental evidence to support that connection. But, there is obviously much missing. Real life-changing NDEs, where people spiritually separate from their bodies and afterward can verify details they would not have any human and plausible way of gathering, are as yet unexplained and cannot be simply attributed to a dying brain, REM activity, anoxia, hallucinations, or sudden bursts of brain electrical activity.

WHAT DO I CONCLUDE?

In my case, being both a physician and scientist, I have approached what I experienced with some trepidation. What is clear to me is that my consciousness survived death and I was able to verify details of my NDE, which as usual included an out-of-body experience, that I would have no conceivable way of knowing except through conscious travel and existence of my spiritual self outside of my brain and body. As Robin Kelly, MD, states, "Our brain may not be the seat of consciousness, but merely a vessel through which consciousness is realized."[30]

I can only hope that, through further experimentation and study, meaningful data will be found to corroborate what many of us near-death experiencers already know—that the gift of life is greater than the sum of its parts and, whatever consciousness is, survives death.

CHAPTER SEVEN

Near-Death Experiences Evidence for Their Reality

Jeffrey Long, MD

The combination of nine lines of evidence converge on the conclusion that near-death experiences are medically inexplicable. Any one or several of the nine lines of evidence would likely be reasonably convincing to many, but the combination of all of the presented nine lines of evidence provides powerful evidence that NDEs are, in a word, real.

INTRODUCTION

NEAR-DEATH EXPERIENCES (NDES) ARE REPORTED by about 17% of those who nearly die.[1] NDEs have been reported by children, adults, scientists, physicians, priests, ministers, among the religious and atheists, and from countries throughout the world. Several are reported in this book.

While no two NDEs are the same, there are characteristic features that are commonly observed in NDEs. These characteristics include a perception of seeing and hearing apart from their physical body; passing into or through a tunnel; encountering a mystical light; intense and generally positive emotions; a review of part or all of one's prior life experiences; encountering deceased loved ones; and a choice to return to an earthly life.[2]

METHODS

There is no uniformly accepted definition of a near-death experience. Definitions of an NDE with some variability have been used throughout the 35 plus years that NDEs have been the subject of scholarly investigation. For my retrospective investigations, an NDE was required to have both a near-death and an experience component.

Individuals were considered to be "near-death" if they were so physically compromised that if their condition did not improve they would be expected to irreversibly die. Near-death experiencers (NDErs) included in my investigations were generally unconscious and may have required cardiopulmonary resuscitation. The "experience" component of an NDE had to occur when those having them were near death. Also, the experience had to be reasonably lucid, which excluded fragmentary or brief disorganized memories. For an experience to be classified as an NDE, it had to register a score of seven or above on the NDE Scale.[3] The NDE Scale asks 16 questions about the NDE content and is the most validated scale to help distinguish NDEs from other types of experiences.

In 1998, a website called the Near Death Experience Research Foundation (NDERF, nderf.org) was established to conduct NDE research and to be a public service. It is NDERF policy that all NDE accounts shared with NDERF are posted on the website should the NDErs grant permission. Nearly all NDErs allow their experiences to be posted on the NDERF website. Portions of the NDERF website, including the NDE questionnaire, have been posted in more than 20 different languages. The NDERF website has consistently been at or near the top of websites listed from a Google search for the term "near-death experiences." This prominence of the NDERF website provided a unique opportunity to conduct a large-scale study of NDEs, including NDEs from around the world. At the current time there are more than 3,700 NDEs posted on the NDERF website, which is by far the largest collection of publicly accessible NDE accounts in the world.

The NDERF website provides a form on which near-death experiencers can share a detailed narrative of their experiences, and includes a detailed questionnaire. Extensive prior studies found that an Internet survey has validity equivalent to traditional pencil-and-paper survey.[4] All experiences shared with the NDERF website are reviewed. Sequentially shared NDEs from the NDERF website were studied. NDEs included for study were single NDE accounts, shared in English, and were shared by the individual who personally had the NDE. An investigation of the NDEs shared with NDERF led to nine lines of evidence suggesting the reality of NDEs.

RESULTS SUGGESTING THE REALITY OF NEAR-DEATH EXPERIENCES

Line of Evidence #1

Lucid, organized experiences while unconscious, comatose, or clinically dead

Near-death experiences occur at a time when persons are so physically compromised that they are typically unconscious, comatose, or clinically dead. Considering NDEs from both a medical perspective and logically, it should not be possible for unconscious people to report highly lucid experiences that are clear and logically structured. Nonetheless most NDErs report supernormal consciousness at the time of their NDEs.

The NDERF survey asked, "How did your highest level of consciousness and alertness during the experience compare to your normal, everyday consciousness and alertness?" Of 1,122 NDErs surveyed, 835 (74.4%) indicated they had "More consciousness and alertness than normal"; 229 (20.4%) experienced "Normal consciousness and alertness"; and only 58 (5.2%) had "Less consciousness and alertness than normal."

The NDERF survey also asked, "If your highest level of consciousness and alertness during the experience was different from your normal everyday consciousness and alertness, please explain." In response to this question, NDErs commonly reported that consciousness during their experiences was "clear," "more aware," and often associated with heightened awareness.

Near-death experiences associated with cardiac arrest have been reported in dozens of previously published studies. Over one hundred NDEs occurring during cardiac arrest have been reported in these five studies alone.[5] Prior studies found that 10–20 seconds following cardiac arrest, electroencephalogram measurements generally find no significant measureable brain cortical electrical activity.[6] A prolonged, detailed, lucid experience following cardiac arrest should not be possible, yet this is reported in many NDEs. Cardiac arrest patients are typically amnesic or confused regarding events that occurred immediately prior to or following the cardiac arrest. Three studies illustrate this.[7]

Line of Evidence #2

Seeing ongoing events from a location apart from the physical body while unconscious (out-of-body experience)

A common characteristic of near-death experiences is an out-of-body experience. An out-of-body experience (OBE) is the apparent separation of consciousness from the body. About 45% of near-death experiencers report OBEs that involve them seeing and often hearing ongoing earthly events from a perspective that is apart, and usually above, their physical bodies. Following cardiac arrest, NDErs may see, and later accurately describe, their own resuscitation.

The first prospective study of the accuracy of out-of-body observations during near-death experiences was by Michael Sabom, MD.[8] This study investigated a group of patients who had cardiac arrests with NDEs that included OBEs, and compared them with a control group of patients who experienced cardiac crises but did not have NDEs. Both groups of patients were asked to describe their own resuscitation as best they could. Sabom found that the group of NDE patients was much more accurate than the control group in describing their own resuscitations.

Another prospective study of out-of-body observations during near-death experiences with similar methodology to Sabom's study was published by Penny Sartori, PhD.[9] This study also found that near-death experiencers were often remarkably accurate in describing details of their own resuscitations. The control group that did not have NDEs was highly inaccurate and often could only guess at what occurred during their resuscitations.

Two large retrospective studies investigated the accuracy of out-of-body observations during near-death experiences. The first was by Janice Holden, EdD.[10] Dr. Holden reviewed NDEs with OBEs in all previously published scholarly articles and books, and found 89 case reports. Of the case reports reviewed, 92% were considered to be completely accurate with no inaccuracy whatsoever when the OBE observations were later investigated.

Another large retrospective investigation of near-death experiences that included out-of-body observations was recently published.[11] This study was a review of 617 NDEs that were sequentially shared on the NDERF website. Of these NDEs, there were 287 NDEs that had OBEs with sufficient information to allow objective determination of the reality of their descriptions of their observations during the OBEs. Review of the 287 OBEs found that 280 (97.6%) of the OBE descriptions were entirely realistic and lacked any content that seemed unreal. In this group of 287 NDErs with OBEs, there were 65 (23%) who personally investigated the accuracy of their own OBE observations after recovering from their life-threatening event. Based on these later investigations, none of these 65 OBErs found any inaccuracy in their own OBE observations.

The high percentage of accurate out-of-body observations during near-death experiences does not seem explainable by any possible physical brain function as it is currently known. This is corroborated by OBEs during NDEs that describe accurate observations while they were verifiably clinically comatose.[12] Further corroboration comes from the many NDEs that have been reported with accurate OBE observations of events occurring far from their physical body, and beyond any possible physical sensory awareness.[13] NDERF has received scores of NDEs with OBE observations during NDEs containing highly unexpected observations that were later confirmed as factual. An illustrative example was an NDE with an OBE in which the patient described the cardiac surgeon "flapping his arms as if trying to fly." The surgeon later verified this, stating that after scrubbing in he flattened his hands on his chest to keep them sterile and was rapidly pointing with his elbows to give instructions. NDE accounts have been reported with OBEs that accurately observed events that were completely unexpected by the NDErs.[14] This further argues against NDEs as being a result of illusory memories originating from what the NDErs might have expected during a close brush with death.

Line of Evidence #3

Near-death experiences with vision in the blind and supernormal vision

There have been a few case reports of near-death experiences in the blind. The largest study of this was by Kenneth Ring, PhD.[15] This investigation included 31 blind or substantially visually impaired individuals who had NDEs or out-of-body experiences. Of the 31 individuals in the study, 10 were not facing life-threatening events at the time of their experiences, and thus their experiences were not NDEs. There were 14 individuals who were blind from birth in this study, and nine of them described vision during their experiences. This investigation presented case reports of those born totally blind that described NDEs that were highly visual with content consistent with typical NDEs.

The NDERF website has received additional case reports of near-death experiences among those functionally and/or legally blind. For illustration, the following NDE happened to Marta, a five-year-old blind girl who walked into a lake:

"I slowly breathed in the water and became unconscious. A beautiful lady dressed in bright white light pulled me out. The lady looked into my eyes and asked me what I wanted. I was unable to think of anything until it occurred to me to travel around the lake. As I did so, I saw detail that I would not have seen in "real" life. I could go anywhere, even to the tops of trees, simply by my intending to go there. I was legally blind. For the first time I was able to see leaves on trees, bird's feathers, bird's eyes, details on telephone poles and what was in people's back yards. I was seeing far better than 20/20 vision."[16]

An NDERF survey question asked 1,122 near-death experiencers, "Did your vision differ in any way from your normal, everyday vision (in any aspect, such as clarity, field of vision, colors, brightness, depth perception degree of solidness/transparency of objects, etc.)?" In response, 722 (64.3%) answered "Yes," 182 (16.2%) said "Uncertain," and 218 (19.4%) responded "No." A review of narrative responses to this question revealed that vision during NDEs was often apparently supernormal. Here are some illustrative examples from NDEs:

> "Colors were beyond any I had ever seen."
> "Everything seemed so much more colorful and brighter than normal."
> "My vision was greatly increased. I was able to see things as close or as far as I needed. There was no strain involved it was almost like auto zooming a camera."
> "I had 360 degree vision, I could see above, below, on my right, on my left, behind, I could see everywhere at the same time!"

Vision in near-death experiencers who are blind, including those totally blind from birth, has been described in many case reports. This, along with the finding that vision in NDEs is usually different from normal everyday vision and often described as supernormal, further suggests that NDEs cannot be explained by our current understanding of brain function. This is also further evidence that NDEs are not a product of what NDErs would have expected to occur during a life-threatening event.

Line of Evidence #4

Near-death experiences that occur while under general anesthesia

Under adequate general anesthesia it should not be possible to have a lucid organized memory. Prior studies using EEG and functional imaging of the brains of patients under general anesthesia provide substantial evidence that the anesthetized brain should be unable to produce lucid memories.[17, 18] As previously discussed, following cardiac arrest the EEG becomes flat in 10 to 20 seconds, and there is usually amnesia prior to and following the arrest. The occurrence of a cardiac arrest while under general anesthesia is a combination of circumstances in which no memory from that time should be possible. Here is an illustrative example of an NDE that occurred under general anesthesia during surgery for a heart valve replacement:

> During my surgery I felt myself lift from my body and go above the operating table. The doctor told me later that they had kept my heart open and stopped for a long time, and they had a great amount of difficulty getting my heart started again. That must have been when I left my body because I could see the doctors nervously trying to get my heart going. It was strange to be so detached from my physical body. I was curious about what they were doing but not concerned. Then, as I drifted farther away, I saw my father at the head of the table. He looked up at me, which did give me a surprise because he had been dead now for almost a year.[19]

I reviewed 613 near-death experiences shared with NDERF, and found 23 NDEs that appeared to have occurred while under general anesthesia. Cardiac arrest was the most common life-threatening event that was described in association with the occurrence of these NDEs. I compared the responses of these 23 NDErs to the 590 non-anesthesia NDErs by reviewing how both groups responded to 33 survey questions that asked about the content of the NDEs.

Chi-square statistics was used for this comparison. Due to the large number of questions asked, statistical significance was set at $p \leq .01$. The only statistically significant difference between the two groups was that the anesthesia NDEs were more likely to describe tunnels in their experiences.

An NDERF survey question asked, "How did your highest level of consciousness and alertness during the experience compare to your normal everyday consciousness and alertness?" For the NDEs occurring under general anesthesia, 19 (83%) of the respondents answered, "More consciousness and alertness than normal," to this question, compared to 437 (74%) for all other NDEs. The responses to this question by the two groups were not statistically significantly different. This suggests, remarkably, that the level of consciousness and alertness in NDEs is not modified by general anesthesia.

Other near-death experience investigators have reported NDEs occurring while under general anesthesia. Bruce Greyson, MD, a leading NDE researcher at the University of Virginia, states:

> In our collection of NDEs, 127 out of 578 NDE cases (22%) occurred under general anesthesia, and they included such features as OBEs that involved experiencers' watching medical personnel working on their bodies, an unusually bright or vivid light, meeting deceased persons, and thoughts, memories, and sensations that were clearer than usual.[20]

NDEs due to cardiac arrest while under general anesthesia occur and are medically inexplicable.

Line of Evidence #5

Near-death experiences and life reviews

Some near-death experiences include a review of part or all of their prior lives. This NDE element is called a life review. NDErs typically describe their life review from a third-person perspective. The life review may include awareness of what others were feeling and thinking at the time earlier in their life when they interacted with them. This previously unknown awareness of what other people were feeling or thinking when they interacted with them is often surprising and unexpected to the NDErs. Here is an example of a life review:

> I went into a dark place with nothing around me, but I wasn't scared. It was really peaceful there. I then began to see my whole life unfolding before me like a film projected on a screen, from babyhood to adult life. It was so real! I was looking at myself, but better than a 3-D movie as I was also capable of sensing the feelings of the persons I had interacted with through the years. I could feel the good and bad emotions I made them go through.[21]

In my review of 617 near-death experiences from NDERF, a life review occurred in 88 NDEs (14%). None of the life reviews in these NDEs appeared to have any unrealistic content as determined by my review or based on comments by the NDErs about their own life reviews. Life reviews may include long-forgotten details of their earlier life that the NDErs later confirm really happened. If NDEs were unreal experiences, it would be expected that there would be significant error in life reviews and possibly hallucinatory features. The consistent accuracy of life reviews, including the awareness of long-forgotten events and awareness of the thoughts and feelings of others from past interactions, further suggests the reality of NDEs.

Line of Evidence #6

Encountering deceased loved ones in near-death experiences

Near-death experiencers may describe encounters with people that they knew during their earthly life. The following is an example of encountering a deceased loved one in an NDE. This example is also notable as the NDEr was born totally deaf:

> I approached the boundary. No explanation was necessary for me to understand, at the age of ten, that once I cross[ed] the boundary, I could never come back—period. I was more than thrilled to cross. I intended to cross, but my ancestors over another boundary caught my attention. They were talking in telepathy, which caught my attention. I was born profoundly deaf and had all hearing family members, all of which knew sign language! I could read or communicate with about twenty ancestors of mine and others through telepathic methods. It overwhelmed

me. I could not believe how many people I could telepathize with simultaneously.[22]

When people known to the near-death experiencers are encountered in NDEs, the great majority are people who are deceased. A study by Emily Kelly, PhD, was a comparison of 74 NDEs with descriptions of encountering deceased individuals with 200 NDEs that did not describe encounters with the deceased.[23] This study found that when NDErs encountered beings known to them from their earthly lives in their NDEs, only 4% described meeting beings that were alive at the time of their experiences. I reviewed 84 NDEs from NDERF that described encounters with individual(s) that they knew in their earthly life.[24] There were only three NDEs (4%) where the encountered beings were alive at the time of the NDEs, consistent with the findings of the Kelly study.

In dreams or hallucinations when familiar persons are present they are much more likely to be living and from recent memory.[25] This is in sharp contrast to near-death experiences in which familiar persons encountered are almost always deceased. Cases have been reported by NDErs of seeing a person whom they thought was living, but in fact had recently died.[25,26] These cases illustrate that NDEs cannot be explained by the experiencer's expectation of what would happen during a life-threatening event. Further evidence that NDEs are not a result of expectation comes from the aforementioned Kelly study where in one-third of the cases the encountered deceased person had a poor or distant relationship with the NDEr, or was someone that had died before the NDEr was born.[23]

Line of Evidence #7

Near-death experiences of young children

Investigation of near-death experiences in very young children is important because at an early age they are less likely to have established religious beliefs, cultural understandings about death, or even an awareness of what death is. Very young children would be very unlikely to have heard about near-death experiences or understand them. I investigated the NDEs in children age five and younger in the same group of 613 NDErs previously discussed in the section on NDEs while under general anesthesia. Two NDErs were excluded as they did not provide their age in the survey. The study groups included 26 NDErs who were age 5 and younger (average 3.6 years old) and 585 NDErs age 6 and older at the time of their NDEs. The NDERF survey included 33 questions about the content of their NDEs. Chi-square statistics were used to compare the responses to these 33 questions between the two groups.[27] There was no statistically significant difference to the responses between the two groups to any of the 33 questions. The NDERF study found that the content of NDEs in children age five and younger appeared to be the same as the content of NDEs in older children and adults. The findings of the NDERF study are corroborated by the investigation of Cherie Sutherland, PhD, who reviewed thirty years of scholarly literature regarding the NDEs of children and concluded:

> It has often been supposed that the NDEs of very young children will have a content limited to their vocabulary. However, it is now clear that the age of children at the time of their NDE does not in any way determine its complexity. Even pre-linguistic children have later reported quite complex experiences. . . . Age does not seem in any way to affect the content of the NDE.[28]

Very young children have near-death experience content that is strikingly similar to that of older children and adults. This is further evidence that NDEs are occurring independently of preexisting cultural beliefs, religious training, or awareness of the existence of NDE.

Line of Evidence #8

Cross-cultural study of near-death experiences

Portions of the NDERF website, including the questionnaire, have been translated into 23 different languages. Over 500 near-death experiences in non-English languages have been shared with NDERF over the years. Dozens of volunteers have translated the non-English NDEs into English. Both the non-English and English translated versions of the NDEs are posted on the NDERF website. Over 60,000 people currently visit the NDERF website each month. Many website visitors are bilingual, and this helps assure that the NDEs are accurately translated.

My investigation of NDEs from around the world that have been translated into English contain strikingly similar content.[29] If near-death experiences were considerably influenced by pre-existing religious and cultural beliefs, it would be expected that there would be significant differences in the content of NDEs from different cultures around the world. However, in my review of over 500 NDEs from dozens of countries around the world I found impressive similarities in the content of these NDEs.

I investigated 19 non-Western NDEs, where a "non-Western country" was defined as an area of the world that are not predominantly of Jewish or Christian heritage.[30] These 19 non-Western NDEs were compared to a group of NDEs shared in English from Western countries that were predominantly English speaking. This investigation concluded:

> All near-death experience elements appearing in Western NDEs are present in non-Western NDEs. There are many non-Western NDEs with narratives that are strikingly similar to the narratives of typical Western NDEs. At a minimum, it may be concluded that non-Western NDEs are much more similar to Western NDEs than dissimilar.[31]

Two recent investigations of Muslim near-death experiences in non-Western countries have been reported. An investigation of 19 Iranian Muslim NDEs concluded:

> Our results suggest that Muslim NDEs may actually be quite common, as they are in the West, and may not be especially different in their key features from Western NDEs and therefore not heavily influenced by cultural variations, including prior religious or spiritual beliefs.[32]

Another study of eight Muslim NDEs found:

> Although the documentation standard of the available cases is generally low, these accounts indicate that structure and contents of NDEs from

many non-Western Muslim communities are largely similar to those reported in the Western NDE literature.[33]

The lack of significant differences in the content of near-death experiences around the world, including NDEs from non-Western countries, suggests that NDE content is not substantially modified by preexisting cultural influences. This finding is consistent with the previously discussed finding that children age five and under, who during their brief lives have received far less cultural influence than adults, have NDEs with content that is essentially the same as older children and adults. Other common forms of altered consciousness, such as dreams or hallucinations, are much more likely to be significantly influenced by prior cultural beliefs and life experiences. The lack of significant differences in the content of NDEs around the world is consistent with the concept that NDEs occur independently from physical brain function as currently understood.

Line of Evidence #9

Near-death experience aftereffects

Following near-death experiences significant changes in the lives of NDErs are commonly observed. The most recent version of the NDERF survey asked NDErs, "My experience directly resulted in . . . :"

The responses of 278 NDErs to the question were:

Large changes in my life	152	54.7 %
Moderate changes in my life	68	24.5 %
Slight changes in my life	28	10.1 %
No changes in my life	14	5.0 %
Unknown	16	5.8 %

Changes in beliefs and values following near-death experiences are often called aftereffects. Given that a life-threatening event without an NDE might result in life changes, some of the best evidence for NDE-specific aftereffects came from the largest prospective NDE study ever reported. This study, conducted by Pim van Lommel, MD, divided survivors of cardiac arrest into a group that had NDEs and a group that did not.[12] The aftereffects of both groups were assessed two and eight years after the cardiac arrests. The group of cardiac arrest survivors with NDEs were statistically more likely to have a reduced fear of death, increased belief in life after death, increased interest in the meaning of life, acceptance of others, and greater love and empathy for others. It may take years after NDEs for the aftereffects to become fully manifest. The aftereffects may be so substantial that NDErs may seem to be very different people to their loved ones and family. The consistency, intensity, and durability of NDE aftereffects are consistent with the NDErs' typical personal assessments that their experiences were very meaningful and significant. It is remarkable that NDEs often occur during only minutes of unconsciousness, yet commonly result in substantial and life-long transformations of beliefs and values.

CONCLUSION OF STUDY

Multiple lines of evidence point to the conclusion that near-death experiences are medically inexplicable and cannot be explained by known physical brain function. Many of the preceding lines of evidence would be remarkable if they were reported by a group of individuals during conscious experiences. However, NDErs are generally unconscious or clinically dead at the time of their experiences and should not have any lucid organized memories from their time of unconsciousness.

It is informative to consider how near-death experiencers themselves view the reality of their experiences. An NDERF survey of 1,122 NDErs asked "How do you currently view the reality of your experience?" and received the following responses:

Experience was definitely real	962	95.6 %
Experience was probably real	40	4.0 %
Experience was probably not real	3	0.3 %
Experience was definitely not real	1	0.1 %

The great majority of more than 1,000 near-death experiencers believed that their experiences were definitely real. The 1,122 NDErs surveyed included many physicians, scientists, attorneys, and nurses. These findings suggest that, for the majority of us who have not personally experienced an NDE, we should be very cautious about labelling NDEs as "unreal." Given that such a high percentage of NDErs consider their experiences to be "definitely real," it would be reasonable to accept their assessment of the reality of their personal experience short of good evidence to the contrary.

After more than 35 years of scholarly investigation of near-death experience, the totality of what is observed in NDEs has not been adequately explained based on physical brain function. It is beyond the scope of this chapter to review the many proposed "explanations" of near-death experience. They can be found elsewhere in this book. Over the years, there have been more than 20 different "explanations" of NDE suggested that cover the gamut of physiological, psychological, and cultural causes. If any one or several of these "explanations" were widely accepted as plausible, then there would be no need for so many different "explanations" of NDE. Among those who believe that physical brain function must explain everything that is experienced in all NDEs, there is no consensus whatsoever about how physical brain function produces NDEs.

SUMMARY

The combination of the preceding nine lines of evidence converges on the conclusion that near-death experiences are medically inexplicable. Any one or several of the nine lines of evidence would likely be reasonably convincing for many scientists, but the combination of all of the presented nine lines of evidence provides powerful evidence that NDEs are, in a word, real.

CHAPTER EIGHT

Apparently Non-Physical Veridical Perception in Near-Death Experiences

Janice Miner Holden, EdD

Apparently non-physical veridical perception has been documented in many cases, including as a result of prospective hospital studies of psychological experiences during cardiac arrest, but has so far eluded documentation under controlled hospital study conditions.

BEGINNING WITH PSYCHIATRIST RAYMOND MOODY'S 1975 book *Life After Life*[1] that was most instrumental in opening the contemporary field of near-death studies, near-death experience (NDE) researchers and investigators have documented cases of veridical perception. In these cases, individuals who survived a close brush with death with an NDE reported perceptions during their NDEs that were subsequently corroborated as accurate. Most intriguing were cases in which, based on the condition and position of the experiencer's (NDEr's) physical body at the time of the NDE, as well as current models of perceptual processes, and ruling out the likelihood that the NDEr could have arrived at the perception through a process of deduction based on probability, expectation, and/or information leakage from purposeful or inadvertent sources, the NDEr should not have been able to perceive what the NDEr reported having perceived. Nevertheless, that perception was found to be accurate and correct. I termed these cases "*apparently non-physical veridical perception*"(AVP).[2] What makes these cases particularly interesting is that they brought unique data to a fundamental question regarding NDEs. NDErs are typically adamant that their NDEs were real or hyperreal, but beyond this subjective reality, might NDEs also be objectively real?

Researchers have established clearly that NDEs are phenomenologically different from dreams and hallucinations, including that they appear to reflect an underlying structure.[3,4] Nevertheless, variations in perceptions during NDEs indicate that at least some content of each experience is unique to the individual. For example, in a brief analysis of visions of the Christian figure, Jesus, in NDEs posted at the Near-Death Experience Foundation website (www.nderf.org), I found that various NDErs described his appearance differently. Some changes might be explainable, such as different clothing, but other features that would presumably be consistent varied from NDEr to NDEr. For example, Jesus's physical build was described variously as slender, healthy and robust, or strong and powerful; his height as nothing exceptional, 6'1.5", 6'5", and tall as a ceiling; his skin color as quite dark, olive-brown, like brass, copper, and suntan; his eye color dark brown, light brown with flecks of amber, burning liquid gold, blue, piercing blue, and like flames of fire; and his voice was absent due to telepathic communication, very soft, almost musical, like thunder but louder, and like a freight train, almost deafening. However, the presence of perceptual variations does not preclude the possibility that at least some perceptions in NDEs might be veridical.

Similar to cardiologist and pioneering NDE researcher Michael Sabom[5] but using different terminology, I have conceptualized near-death experiences as comprised of three aspects related to what the NDEr perceives: 1. nonmaterial, 2. material, and 3. transmaterial.[2] In the nonmaterial aspect, the NDEr experiences a peaceful, floating sensation without respect to their physical body; there is no perception of either material or transmaterial phenomena and no clear sense of consciousness either being or not being associated with their physical body—hence the term "nonmaterial."

In the material aspect, the NDEr perceives their consciousness to be functioning—typically lucidly or hyper-lucidly—at a location apart from their physical body, most commonly above the body but including even locations remote from it. From this location, the NDEr perceives the material, physical world, although attempts to interact with the material world typically fail, such as trying to communicate verbally with a living person or reaching out to touch a living person and finding their "hand" passes through her or him, in either case without an indication that the person—either at the time or upon later questioning—sensed anything.

In the transmaterial aspect, the NDEr, again typically with lucidity or hyper-lucidity, perceives phenomena—entities and/or domains—that are not of a material, physical nature. Entities include deceased loved ones (discarnates) and/or spiritual beings, sometimes identifiable religious figures but often unidentifiable yet usually deeply familiar, such as spiritual guides, angelic beings, or, more rarely, demonic entities. Environments include those of exquisite, unearthly beauty in which earth-like phenomena have unearthly characteristics such as sentience in every blade of grass; they also include structure-like phenomena such as halls of knowledge and cities of light; again, more rarely, they include hellish scenes. During the transmaterial aspect the NDEr not only perceives but also interacts with transmaterial phenomena, most often involving mind-to-mind communication with entities.

Readers familiar with the term "out-of-body experience" (OBE) may recognize its similarity to the two latter NDE aspects. Like Sabom,[5] I consider the entire NDE beyond the nonmaterial aspect to be an extended OBE. However, users of that term typically do not differentiate between material and transmaterial content. This distinction is useful, if not important, in the study of AVP—hence my eschewing of the term OBE and using instead my "aspect" terminology.

Although NDErs tend to report that the three aspects occur in the order presented above, they actually can occur in any order, and NDErs sometimes report going back and forth between two or more aspects. In addition, NDErs tend to report these aspects to be distinct from each other, but they sometimes have reported the material and transmaterial to co-occur, as in the case of Tricia, whom I interviewed in 2008. She reported that after her devastating car accident one morning, physicians told her and her family that because of extensive spinal damage she would never walk again. In surgery that evening she went into cardiac arrest and suddenly found her consciousness functioning lucidly outside of her body, observing the operating room. Behind each of the two surgeons was a spiritual entity with whom Tricia communicated mind-to-mind via light from the beings' eyes. At one point, they transmitted light into the surgeons' bodies and, through them, into Tricia's physical body—which Tricia understood to mean that she would heal and walk again. When I again interviewed her years later she was completely ambulatory. Her NDE illustrates how, in some NDEs, material and transmaterial phenomena can not only co-occur but also interact. It is because the aspects do not always occur in sequence and because they are not always distinct that I refer to them as "aspects" rather than as "phases" or "stages."

Because the nonmaterial aspect involves no phenomena beyond a peaceful, floating sensation, AVP does not occur in that aspect. However, it has been reported in the other two aspects. The earliest example I have found was that of physician A. S. Wiltse,[6] who published a report of his own AVP that Frederic W. H. Myers[7] subsequently investigated. A recent example of AVP during the material aspect was reported in a documentary by an anesthetist and intensive care physician from Toulouse, France, Jean Jacques Charbonier:

> Narrator: *A change in the mentality of healthcare professionals can be seen. Is it the result of the studies carried out by a growing number of researchers around the world, or are there simply more people verifying the detailed perceptions of their patients when they come out of the anesthetic?*
> Charbonier [narrator providing English-translated voiceover]: *I operated on a woman under general anesthetic, and when she woke up, she described her operation as if she had been on the ceiling. Not only that, she also described the operation that took place in the next theater: the amputation of a leg. She saw the leg; she saw them put the leg in a yellow bag. She couldn't possibly have invented that—and she described it as soon as she woke up.* [footage of an operating room with a large yellow medical waste bag] *I checked afterwards, and the operation had, indeed, taken place in the next theater. A leg had been amputated at the very same time that she was under anesthetic and, thus, totally disconnected from the world.*[8]

AVP also has purportedly occurred during the transmaterial aspect of NDEs. In orthopedist Mary Neal's[9] NDE associated with a drowning incident, an entity she identified as Jesus told her that her son would die by his eighteenth birthday. Ten years later as that date approached, she had a dream indicating a possible reprieve from this fate. However, shortly after he turned 18—ironically, on the day she had submitted the final manuscript of her book describing her NDE—she received the phone call in which she was informed that while her son and a friend were exercising along the side of a road, he had been hit by a car and had died upon impact.

Beyond a predominantly accurate prediction of an otherwise presumably unforeseeable tragic accident, several cases of transmaterial AVP exist in which the NDEr encountered a discarnate not known to have died. Psychiatrist Bruce Greyson[10] reported several such cases he had gleaned from the professional literature. He included nine examples of the most evidential type of case—in which the discarnate had died just prior to being perceived by the experiencer and, thus, neither the experiencer nor anyone in attendance could have known of the death through normal physical means. Of these nine cases from both near-death experiences and nearing-death (deathbed) visions, four were reported by physicians, including Moody, Elisabeth Kübler-Ross, and K. M. Dale. Greyson included four additional cases reported by physicians in which the experiencer perceived a discarnate unknown to him or her but subsequently verified. A recent example of this latter type—but not reported by a physician—is the case of four-year-old Colton Burpo who perceived in his NDE a sister whom his mother had miscarried—a topic the parents felt confident had never been discussed in the child's presence.[11]

HOSPITAL STUDIES

Cases such as those described above vary in evidential value, and even the most evidential have been the subject of heated debate in the professional literature.[12, 13, 14, 15, 16, 17] To avoid the vulnerability to alternative explanations inherent in cases that occurred under scientifically uncontrolled conditions, several researchers and research teams have attempted to capture AVP under controlled conditions. These researchers focused on the material aspect of NDEs and based their studies on the assumption that "vision" during that aspect is comparable to vision in the physical body, an assumption that was largely substantiated through my doctoral dissertation research.[18]

All six prospective field studies of AVP to date have involved the same basic protocol: conducted in one or more hospitals in rooms in which cardiac arrest would most likely occur; using visual targets visible from the ceiling but not from normal eye level; and monitoring resuscitations from cardiac arrest or other occasions of patient reports of NDEs in order to follow up to determine patient stability and to approach the patient for interview. Beyond this core, methodological controls have varied from study to study.

In the first study of this type at Lutheran General Hospital in Park Ridge, Illinois, I and chaplain Leroy Joesten[19] employed an artist to create eight-inch square pieces of matte board in six different solid colors and to print on them random combinations of one of six numbers and one of six geometric forms. Using a double-blind research design, we mounted a card 18" below ceiling level and facing the ceiling in each corner of each room in the emergency, intensive care, and cardiac care units—using an installation method whereby we did not see the surface of the card. After three months of interviewing resuscitants from cardiac arrest, we had one patient with an NDE—a recent immigrant to the United States with very poor English skills who declined to participate in the study. Joesten continued to monitor for another nine months with no reported NDEs in the targeted areas, at which point we abandoned the study.

In the second study at Hartford Hospital in Hartford, Connecticut, nurse Madelaine Lawrence[20, 21] used a rectangular electronic "running text" sign placed on a high cabinet of the electrophysiology lab and displaying a nonsense phrase such as "The popsicles are in bloom." After one year of this double-blind study, 25 patients had experienced cardiac arrest as part of their medical procedures: None reported a full NDE, and three reported preliminary material aspect NDEs but none with a consciousness located in "visual" range of the sign.

In the third study at Southampton General Hospital in Southampton, England, physician Sam Parnia and colleagues[22, 23] created boards with various figures on the surface and suspended them from the ceilings of the medical, emergency, and cardiac care units. After one year of interviewing all patients resuscitated from cardiac and respiratory arrest, four patients reported NDEs, none of which included a material aspect.

In the fourth study at Morriston Hospital in Swansea, Wales, nurse Penny Sartori[3, 24] used brightly colored day-glow paper with symbols on the surface and placed them atop the cardiac monitor by each patient's bedside. After five years, fewer than eight patients reported NDEs that included a material aspect, and in each case the patient described a consciousness location outside the "visual" range of a target.

In the fifth study at the University of Virginia Hospital in Charlottesville, Virginia, Greyson, I, and J. Paul Mounsey[25] hired a computer graphics artist to create sixty 20-second animations and to program the computer, upon being started, to quasi-randomly select an animation and play it in a continuous loop, interspersed with a report of the current time, for 90 minutes. We duct-taped the open computer to the top of the monitor near the center of a procedure room in the electrophysiology lab. As a medical procedure involving induced cardiac arrest was about to begin, Greyson climbed on a ladder to start the computer, which then proceeded with a 20-second booting process that gave him plenty of time to return to floor level before the animation began displaying. After 90 minutes, the computer turned off and recorded which of the 60 animations had been displayed. After one year of this double-blind procedure and interviews of 25 patients, representing a total of 50 episodes of cardiac arrest and resuscitation, none reported an NDE.

In the sixth and most recent study at 15 hospitals in the US, UK, and Austria, critical care physician Sam Parnia and colleagues[26] compiled images of "nationalistic and religious symbols, people, animals, and major newspaper headlines" and mounted them on 50–100 shelves in each hospital's emergency room and acute medical wards. In 4.5 years of data collection, out of the 330 patients who survived cardiac arrest to the point of hospital discharge (representing 16% of all in-hospital cardiac arrests), 140 patients met criteria for inclusion in the study, agreed to participate, and were interviewed. Of these, 85 patients reported they did not remember any perception or memory from the time of their cardiac arrest, and the remaining 55 reported they did. Of these 55 who were interviewed in depth and completed the NDE Scale[27,28] to establish the presence and depth of an NDE, nine met criteria. Of these, seven patients' NDEs consisted completely of, in my terms, a transmaterial aspect. Both of the patients with material aspect NDEs experienced cardiac arrest outside the areas equipped with shelves holding visual targets; hence, the study yielded no cases of AVP of targets.

However, as in Sartori et al.'s[3,24] previous study, Parnia et al.[26] reported a case of AVP not involving the visual targets. They prefaced the case description by noting that all measurable brain activity ceases within about 20 seconds of cardiac arrest. Here, one of the two material aspect NDE patients with whom the researchers were able to follow up with an in-depth interview, reported:

> The perception of observing events from the top corner of the room [where the patient] continued to experience a sensation of looking down from above. He accurately described people, sounds, and activities from

> his resuscitation. . . . His medical records corroborated his accounts and specifically supported his descriptions and the use of an automated external defibrillator (AED). Based on current AED algorithms, this [use of the AED] likely corresponded with up to 3 min of conscious awareness during [cardiac arrest] and CPR.[26]

Parnia et al.'s[26] determination that accurate perception occurred well into the cardiac arrest counters previous authors' speculations that AVP is actually the result of conjecture and/or of mental processes involved in the losing or regaining of consciousness. They determined that the accurate perceptions occurred during a time with no measurable brain activity.

Parnia et al.[26] found yet another case to add to those of former researchers who conducted systematic study of cognitive/mental experiences and awareness during cardiac resuscitation. In the pioneering prospective hospital study by Sabom and co-investigator Sarah Kreutziger[5], they found six cases in which patients' reports of their memories during cardiopulmonary resuscitation (CPR) were detailed enough to compare to hospital records—and they found the correspondence to be without error. These researchers compared those accounts to accounts of seasoned cardiac patients—only a few of whom had actually experienced CPR—who speculated what would happen during CPR; by contrast to the NDErs' accurate accounts, each of the comparison group member's accounts contained major errors.[5] Even more to the point, Sartori[3] compared the accuracy with which survivors of CPR—both material NDErs and non-NDErs—described their resuscitations. Whereas material NDErs' accounts corresponded accurately to hospital records, 80% of non-NDErs' accounts contained substantial error. A prospective hospital study in the Netherlands by van Lommel and colleagues[29] yielded a case of AVP that has been thoroughly investigated and found not to be explainable by known physical processes.[30] These results point to the conclusion that material NDErs' memories of their resuscitations are not the result of speculative mental construction or other mental processes.

Why, then, has no visual-target hospital study of AVP yielded a case in which an NDEr "saw" a target? Possible factors are many. In Parnia et al.'s[26] largest study to date, only 22% of cardiac arrests occurred in rooms containing targets; although these were the rooms in which NDEs were most likely to occur, they nevertheless constituted only a minority of those rooms.[26] In addition, in hospital studies overall, NDEs have been reported following only about 10% of resuscitations,[4] in Parnia et al.'s[26] study, material-aspect NDEs occurred in only 2% of successful resuscitations. Considering all these data, the likelihood of (a) a successful resuscitation in (b) a marked room involving (c) a material aspect NDE becomes statistically quite rare. Add to that rarity the unpredictability of location of the material NDEr's perceived consciousness; although a ceiling corner is the most commonly reported location, it is not the only one. On top of these factors, even if the visual target were in the material NDEr's line of "vision," would the NDEr notice it? Results of a perusal of AVP accounts and of my own interviews of NDErs suggest that during their NDEs, experiencers tend to perceive material phenomena that are in some way psychologically important to them. Though exceptions to this generality exist, the use of visual targets that hold no salience for NDErs may further reduce the likelihood that an NDEr would notice and recall it. Taken together, these factors indicate that an NDEr in a hospital study of cardiac arrest patients accurately reporting a visual target would be quite exceptional.

SYSTEMATIC STUDY OF CASE MATERIAL

This state of affairs regarding controlled study of AVP leaves humanity, for the moment, with numerous documented cases of AVP. I and others[30] have argued that, notwithstanding their evidential inferiority to results from systematic studies, these cases collectively provide valuable evidence nonetheless. In preparation for a book summarizing the first 30 years of research in the field of near-death studies, I combed available resources for cases prior to 1975 when NDEs first became widely known, cases arising from systematic studies between 1975 and 2006, and case studies published in peer-reviewed or edited sources during those years. I then analyzed them for factors related to their evidential value including whether the AVP was corroborated by the NDEr alone, by a third party according to the NDEr's report, or by an independent third party, and whether the AVP appeared to contain no error whatsoever, minor error (any non-correspondence between AVP and actual physical circumstances), or major error.[2]

In a replication and extension of that study,[31] I asked three other published near-death researchers to independently evaluate the same cases using the same criteria; after an initial rating and consultation, our final inter-rater reliability was 96.9%. In particular, out of 117 cases altogether, we concurred that NDErs' perceptions in 37 material and five transmaterial cases (36% of the total) were completely accurate and corroborated by a third party—indicating the strongest evidential value. In many of these cases, what NDErs perceived either was unexpected or contradicted their expectations—such as the patient from open-heart surgery who was surprised to see that the heart exposed in his chest was shaped like Africa.[5] These cases spanned 19 publications, nine of which included physicians among their authors, indicating their diverse and credible sources. Although we found the great majority of cases to be completely accurate, we also concurred that seven of the 117 cases (6%) involved either minor or major error, a result that should put to rest conjecture of the file-drawer effect whereby authors are presumed to overlook or fail to report cases involving erroneous perception. These results indicate that when numerous cases from credible sources are studied systematically, they can provide substantial support for the conclusion that accurate AVP occurs in NDEs—albeit as a small percentage of total NDEs.

CONCLUSION

Apparently non-physical veridical perception has been documented in many cases, including as a result of prospective hospital studies of psychological experiences during cardiac arrest, but has so far eluded documentation under controlled hospital study conditions. Though Parnia et al.[26] referred to future attempts to conduct prospective hospital research, I find it difficult to imagine what research methodology could succeed if a nearly-five-year study in 15 hospitals did not yield a single case in which an NDEr reported having perceived a visual target. For the time being, the strongest evidence, though not fulfilling the strict scientistic (science as orthodoxy rather than process) requirement of double-blind randomized methodology, rests with careful investigation of cases of AVP. To this end, studies such as Holden et al.[31] and a forthcoming book by Rivas et al.[30] may keep interest and ingenuity alive regarding possible research methodologies, yet to be conceived, that result ultimately in the capture of AVP under controlled conditions.

CHAPTER NINE

Through the Eyes of a Child Near-Death Experiences in the Young

Penny Sartori, *RN, PhD*

Universal acceptance and recognition of NDEs is especially important in children whose developmental process may even be enhanced and have greater stability in adult life if their NDE is acknowledged at the time it is reported.

DESPITE NEAR-DEATH EXPERIENCES (NDES) BEING reported since early in history and being scientifically researched since the 1970s,[1] there is no theory that adequately explains them. There are many misconceptions about NDEs. They are often attributed to hallucinations of a dysfunctional brain. As a result the multitude of life-changing aftereffects, which are an integral part of NDEs, are often overlooked. Since the advent of prospective clinical and hospital research[2] NDEs are now being acknowledged as a common and valid phenomenon by the medical community.

Cases of NDEs that are particularly compelling are those reported by children, especially those who recall NDEs that occurred as early in their life as the time they were born.[3] Researchers who have contributed greatly to the particular area of childhood NDEs include Melvin Morse,[4] Cherie Sutherland,[5] PMH Atwater,[6] Nancy Evans Bush,[7] William Serdahely,[8] Glen Gabbard, and Stuart Twemlow.[9]

Often the descriptive reports of children surprise the parents and other close relatives as highlighted by the following examples.[10] A four-year-old boy experienced a cardiac arrest during surgery. A few months later following his recovery his father asked him what he would like to do for the day. The child replied that he wanted to go to the park. Puzzled by this request, his father asked which park he meant. They had never visited a park where they were living then (an army camp in Berlin). His son replied:

> The one through the tunnel. . . . The one I went to when I was in the hospital. There was a park with lots of children and swings and things, with a white fence around it. I tried to climb over the fence but this man stopped me and said that I wasn't to come yet and he sent me back down the tunnel and I was back in the hospital again.

Astounded his father commented, "As he was only four at the time I cannot believe that he could make this story up."[11]

In recent years highly publicized cases of childhood NDEs have appeared, with two popular books making it to the *New York Times* best seller list[12] and one of those books made into a Hollywood movie.[13] Phenomenologically, reports of childhood NDEs are very similar to those of adult NDEs and may also include meeting angels or pets and sometimes living relatives. One particular distinction is that children are accompanied to the light by a being, often being led by their hand. Initial reports of NDEs in the literature suggested that some components of adult NDEs, such as the life review and distressing NDEs, were absent in childhood cases,[14] but more recent and thorough research has shown this not to be the case.

Children are often very influenced by their surroundings and their peers; yet several documented cases highlight that what the child experienced during their NDE was at variance to their cultural background and the religious images that they had been brought up with.[15] Following their NDE, some children develop a spirituality that is radically different to the religious views that they grew up with.[16] Researchers have also found that despite some retrospective cases being reported many years after the event, when the experiencers are adults, the NDE is not embellished with time.[17]

The following brief summary of a distressing NDE included the void experience which is characteristic of the second category of distressing NDEs classified by Greyson and Bush.[18] The NDE was reported to the author in 2014 by a forty-nine-year-old man named Jeffrey. He was still trying to understand his NDE that had happened in 1977 when he was twelve years old. The NDE occurred when he was shot in the abdomen; the injury destroyed his spleen and shattered a rib. He recalled viewing the scene in what he now realizes was an out-of-body perspective. He then fell backwards into a "black void"and was panicking because he thought it would hurt when he hit the bottom. He later became aware of what he refers to as his "blob," a shapeless, black cloud that at the same time had edges and borders. It was coming for him. At this point he experienced heightened emotions of negativity. He feared and wondered why no one could hear his screams. He was convinced that this is what it was like to be dead.

He healed remarkably quickly from his injuries and was discharged home two weeks later, completely healthy and ready to return to school but was left with aftereffects, also reported by other NDErs, which were difficult to comprehend:

> I was different than everyone; I knew it, felt it, but no way to explain it. Somehow, I had to learn to fit in. I became an expert at finding coping mechanisms for day to day life, and I also developed an odd sense of intuitive awareness.

This intuitive awareness proved very useful in his career in the United States Air Force where split-second judgment saved him and his aircraft on several occasions. He also developed the ability to see auras and feel the energy from other people. He never fully understood the experience or its aftereffects and more than thirty-seven years later was still trying to reconcile with it which is common amongst NDErs.

In the 1980s pediatrician Melvin Morse undertook NDE research after he spoke to a patient he referred to as Katie, a seven-year-old girl who had reported an NDE when she had almost drowned. He later interviewed pediatric patients in the intensive care unit and found that out of twelve patients who had survived cardiac arrest, every one of them had reported at least one component of the NDE,[19] and he estimated that NDEs would be reported by 70% of children who came close to death.[20]

Interestingly, when Morse followed up on thirty of the childhood NDErs over seven years later, he found that in each case they were well balanced physically and mentally, more likely to eat healthily, did better in school, and none were addicted to alcohol or drugs.[21] This seems to be in direct contrast to the findings of Atwater, who found that over half of her sample of childhood NDErs were depressed and over a third of her sample abused alcohol.[22] This is important as it suggests that the fact that in his case Morse acknowledged, and therefore validated, the NDEs close to the time they occurred helped the children affected to understand and constructively integrate their experiences into their lives, which then led to stability in their adult lives. This also suggests it may especially important for medical professionals caring for children to validate an NDE when it occurs both to the child and the parents. Further research should confirm this.

Understanding an NDE can be very puzzling for both children and adults and often children will not seek help, as in the case of Jeffrey. The aftereffects of unacknowledged NDEs can hinder the integration and understanding of the experience. The less pleasurable consequences of an NDE can manifest as feelings of isolation, estrangement from peer group, and no longer sharing common interests of friends, all of these factors potentially affecting the developmental process of young children. Sutherland[23] emphasizes that believing children when they report their NDE is crucial for their personal growth and change following the NDE, as well as integrating the experience into their life. To restate, it is essential that healthcare workers are educated about NDEs and that there are modifications in practice that ensure not only that NDEs are recognized but that patients are provided with the necessary support to understand them.

NDEs cannot be explained within the current reductionist belief system of consciousness as a byproduct of the brain. The results of prospective research have also ensured that NDEs can no longer be explained away but have to be taken seriously in order to provide essential aspects of patient care. The cases of very young children demonstrate that NDEs can occur when the brain is not fully developed, which also suggests that the NDE can occur independently of a functioning and/or mature brain. This leads to the conclusion that it would be logical to revise the dated concept of consciousness being produced by the brain and explore consciousness from alternative perspectives. Universal acceptance and recognition of NDEs is especially important in children whose developmental process may even be enhanced and have greater stability in adult life if their NDE is acknowledged at the time it is reported.

CHAPTER TEN

Distressing Near-Death Experiences
The Basics

Nancy Evans Bush, MA & Bruce Greyson, MD

Distressing NDEs occur under the same wide range of circumstances and feature most of the same elements as pleasant NDEs. What differs is the emotional tone, which ranges from fear through terror to, in some cases, guilt or despair.

THE GREAT MAJORITY OF NEAR-DEATH experiences (NDEs) reported publicly over the past four decades have been described as pleasant, even glorious. Almost unnoticed in the euphoria about them has been the sobering fact that not all NDEs are so affirming. Some are deeply disturbing.

Few people are forthcoming about such an event; they hide; they disappear when asked for information; if inpatient, they are likely to withdraw; they are under great stress. What do their physicians need to know to deal with these experiences?

VARIETIES OF DISTRESSING NEAR-DEATH EXPERIENCES

We have documented three types of distressing NDEs (DNDEs): inverse, void, and hellish.[1] The brief descriptions below illustrate the types. All examples are from the authors' files unless otherwise indicated.

INVERSE NDE

In some inverse NDEs, features usually reported in other NDEs as pleasurable are perceived as hostile or threatening. A man thrown from his horse found himself floating at treetop height, watching emergency medical technicians working over his body. "No! No! This isn't right!" He screamed, "Put me back!"

But they did not hear him. Next he was shooting through darkness toward a bright light, flashing past shadowy people who seemed to be deceased family members waiting. He was panic-stricken by the bizarre scenario and his inability to affect what was happening.

A woman in childbirth felt her spirit separate from her body and fly into space at tremendous speed, then saw a small ball of light rushing toward her: "It became bigger and bigger as it came toward me. I realized that we were on a collision course, and it terrified me. I saw the blinding white light come right to me and engulf me."

A woman collapsed from hyperthermia and began re-experiencing her entire life: "I was filled with such sadness and experienced a great deal of depression."

THE VOID DNDE

An NDE of the "void" is an ontological encounter with a perceived vast emptiness, often a devastating scenario of aloneness, isolation, sometimes annihilation. A woman in childbirth found herself abruptly flying over the hospital and into deep, empty space. A group of circular entities informed her she never existed, that she had been allowed to imagine her life but it was a joke; she was not real. She argued with facts about her life and descriptions of Earth. "No," they said, "none of that had ever been real; this is all there was." She was left alone in space.[2, pp. 1–5]

Another woman in childbirth felt herself floating on water, but at a certain point, "It was no longer a peaceful feeling; it had become pure hell. I had become a light out in the heavens, and I was screaming, but no sound was going forth. It was worse than any nightmare. I was spinning around, and I realized that this was eternity; this was what forever was going to be. . . . I felt the aloneness, the emptiness of space, the vastness of the universe, except for me, a mere ball of light, screaming."

A woman who attempted suicide felt herself sucked into a void: "I was being drawn into this dark abyss, or tunnel, or void. . . . I was not aware of my body as I know it. . . . I was terrified. I felt terror. I had expected nothingness; I expected the big sleep; I expected oblivion; and I found now that I was going to another plane . . . and it frightened me. I wanted nothingness, but this force was pulling me somewhere I didn't want to go, but I never got beyond the fog."

A man who was attacked by a hitchhiker felt himself rise out of his body: "I suddenly was surrounded by total blackness, floating in nothing but black space, with no up, no down, left, or right. . . . What seemed like an eternity went by. I fully lived it in this misery. I was only allowed to think and reflect."

HELLISH DNDE

Overtly hellish experiences may be the least common type of distressing NDE. A man in heart failure felt himself falling into the depths of the Earth. At the bottom was a set of high, rusty gates, which he perceived as the gates of hell. Panic-stricken, he managed to scramble back up to daylight.

A woman was being escorted through a frighteningly desolate landscape and saw a group of wandering spirits. They looked lost and in pain, but her guide indicated she was not allowed to help them.

An atheistic university professor with an intestinal rupture experienced being maliciously pinched, then torn apart by malevolent beings.[3]

A woman who hemorrhaged from a ruptured Fallopian tube reported an NDE involving "horrific beings with gray gelatinous appendages grasping and clawing at me. The sounds of their guttural moaning and the indescribable stench still remain 41 years later. There was no benign Being of Light, no life video, nothing beautiful or pleasant."

A woman who attempted suicide felt her body sliding downward in a cold, dark, watery environment: "When I reached the bottom, it resembled the entrance to a cave, with what looked like webs hanging. . . . I heard cries, wails, moans, and the gnashing of teeth. I saw these beings that resembled humans, with the shape of a head and body, but they were ugly and grotesque. . . . They were frightening and sounded like they were tormented, in agony."

THREE TYPES OF RESPONSE

These NDEs are traumatic in their realness, their rupturing the sense of worldly reality, and the power of the questions they raise. Three common responses cut across all experience types: the turnaround; reductionism; and the long haul.[2]

1. The Turnaround: "I needed that."

A classic response to profound spiritual experience is conversion, not necessarily changing one's religion but in the original sense of the Latin *convertere* meaning "to turn around." The terrifying NDE is interpreted as a warning about unwise or wrong behaviors, and the need to turn one's life around: "I was being shown that I had to shape up or ship out, one or the other. In other words, 'get your act together,' and I did just that."[4, p. 46]

Movement toward a dogmatic religious community is common in this group. Clinical social worker Kimberly Clark Sharp observed, "All the people I know who have had negative experiences have become Bible-based Christians. . . . They might express it in various sects. But they all feel that they have come back from an awful situation and have a second chance."[5, p. 85]

Fear may remain a powerful influence, but a strict theology may offer a way out. The atheistic professor above who experienced being maliciously pinched, then torn apart by malevolent beings, left his university and attended seminary.[3] Others also reported newfound devotion, "I've stopped drugs, moved back to Florida, and now I'm in Bible college. I used to have a casual attitude toward death, but now I actually fear it more. So yes, it was a warning. I was permitted another chance to change my behavior on earth. . . . I've taken my fear of death and given it to the scriptures."[4, p. 43] Since then, I have dedicated my life to the most high God Jehovah, and spend 60 hours a month speaking and teaching about the Creator of Heaven and Earth and all living creatures. I'm not worried now about when I die, because now I know that God has promised us something far more."

2. Reductionism: "It was only . . ."

As a response to a distressing experience, reductionism has been described as the "defense [that] allows one to repudiate the meaning of an event which does not fit into a safe category" and to "treat the event as if it did not matter."[6, p. 35]

A woman whose anaphylactic reaction precipitated an NDE with both loving and frightening elements concluded,

> There are actual rational explanations for what I experienced. . . . The brain, under stress, releases natural opiates that stop pain and fear. . . . Lack of oxygen disrupts the normal activity of the visual cortex. . . . Too much neural activity in the dying brain causes stripes of activity. . . . Our eyes, even closed, interpret those stripes of activity as . . .

> the sensation of moving forward in a tunnel. . . . There are more brain cells concentrated in the middle of the cortex than on the edges so as we get closer to death, the brain interprets all those dense cells with their crazy activity as a bright light in the middle of our visual field. It's all very scientific.[7, p. 95]

Her conclusion is that, based on the scientific evidence, the experience had no ontological meaning. Any lingering anxieties will go unaddressed.

A woman who had a terrifying experience during childbirth likewise dismissed the reality of the experience: "Perhaps it was the effect of the ether and not an NDE." A woman attacked by a lion dismissed the memory of her DNDE as hallucinatory: "I often wonder if, in the shock of the attack, my mind played tricks on me, and that I may have just been unconscious and my brain deprived of oxygen."

A man who for many years had spoken publicly about his radiant NDE had a second experience in which he felt attacked by gigantic, sinister, threatening geometric forms, leaving him with a deep-seated pessimism and terror of dying. Learning that drug-induced hallucinations include geometric forms, he concluded that his second NDE was "only a drug reaction." This may be an appropriate conclusion clinically, but the experience remains. Reductionism provides a temporary buffer to mask questions and anxieties, but does nothing to resolve them.

3. The Long Haul: "What did I do?"

Other experiencers have difficulty comprehending or integrating terrifying DNDEs. These people, years later, still struggle with the existential implications of the DNDE, "I had an experience which has remained with me for 29 years. . . . It has left a horror in my mind and I have never spoken about it until now." And, "After all these years, the nightmare remains vivid in my mind." "For some reason, [31 years later] all the memories are back and vivid. . . . It's like living it all over again, and I don't want to. I thought I had it all resolved and in its place, but I'm having a really bad time trying to put it away this time."

Also, "For the next 50 years, I would try to repress the memory of the black, threatening experience, because it felt so real it continued to be frightening, no matter how old I got." And, "I've been married for 33 years and I do not even discuss the experience with my husband. . . . Yet it is as clear to me today as it was when it happened." Additionally, "I just buried the whole thing as deeply as possible, got very busy in civic affairs, politics. . . . It seems pretty clear to me now, though the specifics aren't in place, that there's some core issue that still needs dealing with."

"I see this vision as flashbacks constantly. I cannot get this out of my head. . . . I still see it in my mind from my own eyes. It has been two years, yet I have never talked about it. My husband does not even know. . . . I want to put this behind me, but am unable."

This group is often of articulate people haunted by the existential dimension of their DNDEs, searching for a cognitively and emotionally grounding explanation. They find a literal reading of the event intellectually unacceptable, but reductionist explanations only assign a cause without addressing meaning. They struggle to make sense of the DNDEs without destroying them (and their trust in the workings of the world) in the process.

More than others, these experiencers appear to enter psychotherapy, some for many years, though without data this observation may indicate nothing other than openness and financial means. Too often physicians prescribe medications to mask questioning and dismiss the DNDE as fanciful or pathological; therapists will not address the matter or leave the client feeling blamed or romanticize spirituality and cannot deal with its dark side; and clergy have no idea what to say or reject the experience outright.

The religious element of their NDE is often an absence:

> "I was filled with a sense of absolute terror and of being past the help of anyone, even God."
> "I looked around me. Consciously searching for . . . God or some other angelic creature, but I was alone."
> "I expected the Lord to be there, but He wasn't. . . I called on God and He wasn't there. That's what scared me."[4, p. 53]

Overwhelmingly, their questions include some variant of "What did I do to deserve this?" or "What are the rules, if the rules I lived by don't work?" Not for a long time, if ever, do they lose their fear of death. The man above attacked by a hitchhiker still struggled with the aftermath, "I've pondered if I was in that hell; will I go back on my death? Was I sent there for something perhaps I'll do in the future, or something I did in the past? . . . I don't believe in a hell, but it was such a strong experience, there is always that underlying uncertainty and trouble and fear."

POSTTRAUMATIC GROWTH

The psychological literature on posttraumatic growth did not exist in the early years of our study of distressing NDEs, so that aspect of response remains underreported. As a growing number of studies make clear, even the most devastating life event, "like the grit that creates the pearl, is often what propels people to become more true to themselves, take on new challenges, and view life from a wider perspective."[8, p. 7] This is a promising and as yet underdeveloped approach for clinicians working with those who report struggling after a distressing NDE.[9]

SEVEN THINGS TO KNOW ABOUT DISTRESSING NEAR-DEATH EXPERIENCES

1. Distressing NDEs occur under the same wide range of circumstances and feature most of the same elements as pleasant NDEs. What differs is the emotional tone, which ranges from fear through terror to, in some cases, guilt or despair. The reports typically lack two elements common in pleasant NDEs: a positive emotional tone and loss of the fear of death.
2. A notorious reluctance to report a distressing NDE may lead to long-lasting trauma for individuals as well as limiting the data on occurrence. A literature review covering thirty years of research concludes that as many as one in five NDEs may be predominantly distressing.[10]
3. The etiology of all such events remains unknown. Despite decades of clinical studies, none so far adequately explains either the cause or function of NDEs. Further, NDEs cross so many clinical circumstances and demographic bases; there is no way to predict who will have what type of NDE. No evidence supports the conventional assumption that "good" people get pleasant NDEs and "bad" people have distressing ones. Saints have reported extremely disturbing NDEs [11, pp. 63–75] while felons and suicide attempters have encountered bliss.[12, pp. 41–44]

4. Pleasant NDEs tend to convey universal messages of compassion that cross religious and philosophical systems. Distressing NDEs typically have less-focused messages but follow the ancient shamanic pattern of suffering/death/resurrection, which in less metaphoric terms can be read as an invitation to self-examination, disarrangement of core beliefs, and rebuilding. In practical terms, a common interpretation of a distressing NDE is that it is a message to turn one's life around.
5. The description of any NDE is shaped by the experiencer's pre-existing mental categories and vocabulary. As example, although the archetype of a benevolent guide is common in NDEs, individuals typically identify the presence according to their own cultural vocabulary. Any report identifying an archetypal individual by name is a perception that may or may not be factually true but cannot be confirmed as such. Understandably, it is facts like these that religious groups and materialists alike may find troubling. Secular Westerners often believe unfoundedly that an NDE indicates a psychotic episode.
6. The primary effect of many NDEs is a powerful and enduring awareness that the physical world is not the full extent of reality. Because this perception runs so deeply counter to Western materialism, and conversely because its implications affect some dogmatic theological teachings, the new conviction commonly overturns experiencers' personal life and social relationships abruptly and permanently.
7. A major challenge for physicians and other scientists dealing with reports of near-death experience is to manage this intrusion of non-materialist religious and philosophical language and understandings into the hard data of clinical thinking. Curiously, it is at the extremes of religious fundamentalism and material scientism that one finds literalism an issue. For fundamentalists, the accounts are believed to be literally, physically actual; for convinced materialists, they must be dismissed as lunacy because a literal, physical actuality is impossible and no alternative concept is acceptable.

Raymond Moody, MD, PhD, in Chapter One of this book, observed, "The best practice for physicians is to stick strictly to clinical and research concerns."[13, p. 371] The post-NDE convictions of patients and their family members with whom physicians must interact are likely to make that a difficult suggestion to follow. Non-judgmental listening may be the most workable alternative.

SUMMARY

Like the better-publicized pleasurable NDEs, distressing near-death experiences are both fascinating and frustrating as altered states of consciousness. Because of the deeply rooted concept of hell in Western culture and its Christian association with eternal physical torment, these experiences pose serious challenges to the individuals who must shape their lives around such a profoundly durable event, and to their families, friends, and physicians. In the absence of clear-cut clinical data and universal cultural views, physicians are advised that neutrality of opinion and careful listening are likely to constitute best professional practice for addressing these difficult, distressing near-death experiences.

CHAPTER ELEVEN

Near-Death Experiences
The Mind-Body Debate & the Nature of Reality

Eben Alexander III, MD

> *In essence, the long-standing presumption that the sheer complexity of the brain somehow leads to the creation of consciousness fails—no one has been able to offer even the most basic explanation about how that might unfold.*

MY NEAR-DEATH EXPERIENCE

As a neurosurgeon with over twenty years' experience in academic neurosurgery, I thought I had a pretty good idea of how the brain and mind worked. I then awoke early in the morning on November 10, 2008, with severe back pain, followed by the worst headache of my life, and a rapid descent into a week-long coma that began with status epilepticus. I recall nothing that happened in my hospital room over the next seven days, but later came to learn many of the medical details of my illness through discussions with physicians who cared for me and by reviewing my medical records and imaging studies.

For reasons that remain obscure, I had contracted a rapidly progressive case of *E. coli* meningoencephalitis. My neurological exams revealed extensive cortical damage, with some brainstem signs (extraocular motor dysfunction) evident that first day. My CT scans revealed global neocortical involvement (none of the eight lobes of my brain was spared)—cerebral edema, profuse sulcal enhancement, and blurring of the gray-white junction. On the third day, my cerebrospinal fluid (CSF) protein was 1,340 mg/dl, my CSF white blood cell count was 4,300 per mm,^{3} and my CSF glucose level was down to 1.0 mg/dl. I was extremely ill, with diminishing chances for survival and virtually no chance for recovery. My physicians never found a cause for my mysterious malady.[1,2]

The last evidence of any "normal" neocortical function was in the first hours in the ER when witnesses heard me cry out "God help me" after hours of nonsensical gibberish and moans (I have no personal memory of this).

Such a rapid descent into coma, combined with the diagnosis of gram-negative bacterial meningitis, signaled at best a 10% probability of survival at the time I presented to the ER.

My meningitis was initially unresponsive to triple intravenous antibiotics, and relentlessly progressed until the seventh day, at which point my physicians estimated my chance of survival had slimmed to 2% and recommended termination of antibiotics due to the hopeless prognosis. My meningitis finally began to subside on that seventh day, as I began the long and arduous process of awakening back to this world.

Initially, I was completely amnesic for my life before coma. I remembered no words, no personal memories of my life, no religious or scientific concepts, and nothing about being human or existing in this universe. I did not recognize dear family members standing around my bedside. All I remembered was where I had just been, in an extraordinary odyssey that seemed to last for months or years—although it had all occurred within the seven days I lay unconscious in the hospital.

Words and language returned over the following hours and days, and childhood and major life memories were restored to me over a week or two. The rest of my prior knowledge, including over twenty years' experience in neurosurgery and all other scientific and intellectual knowledge, returned in layered fashion, quite complete by eight weeks or so after my coma. My physicians continue to be astonished by my miraculous recovery.

Given the extraordinary memories I had of my time deep in coma, the emerging picture of the entire experience proved impossible to explain as a simple brain-based phenomenon (i.e., as a hallucination, dream state, drug effect, or confabulation). Our modern understanding of the role of the neocortex—the outer surface, or human part, of our brains—holds that it is necessary for the detailed construction of consciousness, but the extreme severity of my meningoencephalitis rules out the participation of my neocortex in generating memories during those seven days. Thanks to its preferential destruction of the neocortex, severe meningoencephalitis is, essentially, a perfect model for human death. That fact would nominate the disease for widespread study in brain and consciousness research, save for one problem: it almost always results in death. Almost no one returns to tell the tale.

As my doctors told me soon after my return, my neocortex was too damaged for me to have experienced anything, much less the extraordinary, ultra-real spiritual realms I visited repeatedly deep in my coma. But I knew I had experienced something remarkable, and I wanted to record and analyze that experience as best as possible—I knew that details of my experience might help refine our understanding of the brain, especially the neocortex, and its relationship to the mechanism and phenomenon of consciousness.

As described in detail in my book *Proof of Heaven: A Neurosurgeon's Journey into the Afterlife*,[1] my memories from deep in coma began in a coarse, murky, unresponsive realm, which I labeled the Earthworm's Eye View. In retrospect, I believe this extremely foreboding, subterranean existence was the best consciousness my physical brain could muster while my neocortex was being destroyed by aggressive gram-negative bacteria.

If one had asked me before my coma, "What would be the next step beyond that Earthworm's Eye View in the progression of your severe meningoencephalitis?" I would have assured you the next phase would be one of no awareness at all. I would have been absolutely wrong.

In fact, the next phase was introduced to me by a slowly spinning white light of great clarity, associated with a perfect musical melody. The approaching light opened like a rip in the fabric of that ugly subterranean realm, leading up into an ultra-real valley (the Gateway Valley) filled with light and colors beyond the normal visual spectrum. It seemed so much more real than this earthly realm—fertile and filled with eternally growing plants, blossoms and buds on trees opening in ripe bloom, sparkling waterfalls and mists, dancing souls and swooping angelic choirs above. One does not see with the eyes, nor hear with the ears, in that realm—at times, the observer becomes entire swaths of that realm as a way of learning lessons about it all, even to the point of becoming other beings and groups of beings to feel and know their own knowing—to empathize with them and know them completely. Communication there goes light years beyond our simplistic linear thinking, beyond the bottleneck of linguistically constrained awareness we experience in these physical bodies in the earthly realm.

I had no body image during any part of this journey, but was moving up through that brilliant valley as a speck of awareness on a butterfly wing, accompanied by millions of other swooping and soaring butterflies of indescribable beauty. There was a lovely young woman accompanying me on the butterfly wing, one who never spoke a word, but whose thoughts of unconditional love and assurance came straight into my awareness. She promised me I would be taken care of, that I had nothing to fear, and that I was completely loved by the awe-inspiring Creator of all that is (as are we all). I came to see that unconditional love has the potential to bring infinite healing.

Causal relationships in that realm, even the temporal flow of events there, all occur in what I call "Deep Time," which is much more robust and related to Divine purpose than the events of our lives in the relatively loose temporal causality to which we are accustomed.

I then realized that the chants and hymns emanating from the swooping angelic choirs above were providing yet another portal into higher realms. The lowest (earthly and spiritual) dimensions collapsed down as my awareness entered increasingly refined spiritual realms, finally arriving at what I called the Core—infinite inky blackness, filled to overflowing with the Divine unconditional love of the Creator, and with brilliant light emerging from an orb brighter than a million stars. I was aware of a strong sense of the three of us—a Divine Being beyond all description, the brilliant orb (a translator or interpreter, perhaps?) and my conscious awareness, which by now was joined with all of consciousness throughout the multiverse, transcending a limited personal consciousness. Through wordless conceptual flow, I was informed I was not there to stay. They would teach me many things, but I would be going "back." Since I had lost all my memories of life on Earth, I had no idea what that meant.

The Divine Being and the orb proceeded to demonstrate so much about all of reality: the fundamental role of love and of consciousness or soul in that realm and in all of existence; the constructs of space-time-mass-energy used to build up this physical world; the role of this physical realm as a kind of "soul school" where we learn and exchange lessons of unconditional love, compassion, forgiveness and mercy; the connectedness of all sentient beings, indeed of all consciousness, to all others and to the Divine. As is typical for such extraordinary journeys, the deeper aspects of these teachings far exceed the capacity of human language—which was created to describe earthly scenarios—to do them justice.

When I initially tried to share my stories with my physicians, they firmly reminded me that my neocortex had been too badly damaged to allow for anything more than the most rudimentary of experiences. Certainly my brain could not have generated or received the ultra-real odyssey I was describing. Given how little I remembered about the brain and mind, and of my own illness, I simply believed my doctors' statements that it must have been a "trick of the dying brain."

As I told my older son, Eben IV, who was majoring in neuroscience in college at the time: "It was all way too real to be real." Within days of waking from the coma, he could tell I had been fundamentally transformed. The scientist in me was eager to research what had happened to me, but Eben advised me to write down everything I could remember about the coma journey before reading anything about near-death experiences, physics, or cosmology. I followed his advice and over the next six weeks wrote around 20,000 words describing my experience before allowing myself to delve deeply into the literature on near-death experiences (NDEs), which I had never previously perused.

A MONUMENTAL CHALLENGE TO UNDERSTAND

I sought to explain everything I remembered from coma as a brain-based mechanism. I was prepared to accept my doctors' assertion that it was a "trick of the dying brain," but I was driven to discover what that trick was. The nine best hypotheses, none of which ultimately held up under scrutiny, are outlined in Appendix B in *Proof of Heaven*. My conclusion, after months of analysis with my doctors and other interested colleagues, was that what I'd witnessed really happened—just not in the physical universe, or in my brain.

That conclusion followed an astonishing revelation about the identity of the beautiful companion on the butterfly wing, whose appearance I could remember so well. I knew I had never seen her before my illness, yet the NDE literature consistently shows that such a "guardian angel" should be one who had been crucially important to me in my lifetime.[3–8] Four months after coma, I discovered that she was in fact the birth sister I had never known, who had died two years before I even knew of her existence. That revelation was the catalyst that launched me into a more complete understanding of the reality of my journey.

Concluding that my experience actually happened, but outside of my brain and the physical universe, demanded an extraordinary shift in my worldview. Such a shift was mandatory if I were to move toward any comprehensive understanding of the world that could incorporate my strange experience and begin to explain the vast spectrum of similar experiences reported over the last several thousand years. At the core of it all was the need to more fully refine our understanding of the nature and mechanism of consciousness itself.

THE ENIGMA OF CONSCIOUSNESS

As a neurosurgeon, I was taught that the brain creates consciousness. Consciousness, based on that conventional view, is an illusion manifested by the subatomic particles, atoms, and molecules of the brain all simply following natural laws. The same line of conventional thinking necessarily concludes that we are all acting at the whim of the natural laws governing all of those subatomic particles and their more complex arrangements in molecules and cells of the brain. In other words, none of us actually has free will at all.

To put this challenge in perspective, it is important to point out that the only thing any one of us truly knows to exist is our own consciousness. What we call "the external world" is actually a model constructed in our minds. Conventional neuroscience would remind us that every experience and memory we've ever had is nothing more than the patterns of electrochemical flickering of 100 billion neurons encased in a three-pound gelatinous mass floating in a warm dark bath. Nothing more. A model of reality, and perhaps a mechanism for processing reality, but not reality itself.

Thus the many physicists and cosmologists who claim to be close to defining a "theory of everything" seem woefully premature, given that a far more robust understanding of the phenomenon of consciousness is necessary for any alleged theory about the nature of reality. Only a few recent physicists have actually risen to this challenge, including Roger Penrose, Henry Stapp, Brian Josephson, and Amit Goswami. But the mystery of the measurement problem in quantum mechanics—which says the observer's mind is intricately involved with the physical reality being observed, i.e., that consciousness is fundamental, not an illusion created by the physical brain—drove many of the brilliant founding fathers of quantum mechanics, including Max Planck, Erwin Schrödinger, Louis Debroglie, Sir James Jeans, Werner Heisenberg, Wolfgang Pauli, and Albert Einstein, into mysticism as they sought deeper understanding.

THE HARD PROBLEM OF CONSCIOUSNESS

My quest also illuminated for me the Hard Problem of Consciousness (HPC), arguably the most profound conundrum known to all of human thought. Although the background challenges of the HPC had existed for millennia in the form of the 2,600-year-old Mind-Body Debate, neuroscientists were running headlong into the HPC in the latter decades of the twentieth century. It was finally labeled the Hard Problem of Consciousness by David Chalmers in his brilliant book "The Conscious Mind," published in 1996.[9]

In essence, the longstanding presumption that the sheer complexity of the brain somehow leads to the creation of consciousness fails—no one has been able to offer even the most basic explanation about how that might unfold. One might expect such a fundamental assumption would be well established after the profusion of neuroscience research in recent decades.

The truth is that the more we come to understand the physical workings of the brain, the more we realize it does not create consciousness at all.[10–15] We are conscious in spite of our brain! The brain serves more as a reducing valve or filter, limiting pre-existing consciousness down to the trickle of the illusory "here-now" in which we find ourselves in this physical realm. This idea is revolutionary, but not new; nineteenth-century luminaries including William James and Frederic W. H. Myers advocated for more serious consideration of the filter theory.

To those who recoil at the suggestion that the brain does not create consciousness, I would mention two common clinical observations that support this idea:

1) terminal lucidity (in which elderly demented patients often have oases of great clarity and insight about their lives, often peaking when they are aware of the souls of departed loved ones there to escort them to the other side), and

2) acquired savant syndromes (in which damage to the brain, be it head trauma, stroke, autism, or what have you, reveals a lacuna of super-human mental

function, such as fantastic capabilities for memory of lists, graphic, artistic or musical abilities, calculational abilities, etc.).

This thinking is not new in our modern neuroscientific era. Wilder Penfield, MD, of Montreal, one of the most prominent neurosurgeons of the twentieth century—who probably still holds the record for number of electrical stimulations of the brain in awake patients during his decades-long career treating epilepsy—wrote a book in 1975 summarizing evidence that the mind (and free will) is not created by the brain.[16]

SYNTHESIS OF SCIENCE AND SPIRITUALITY

Thus, the ongoing interpretation of my deep coma experience, and of tens of thousands of similar spiritually transformative experiences over millennia and across the globe, opens the door to a far richer understanding of the nature of reality. The non-locality of consciousness, i.e., that we can know things beyond the ken of our physical senses, is fundamental in the evolving science. Many top-tier scientists are already pursuing this version of truth,[3, 4, 11, 13, 14] one far grander than anything offered by the simplistic materialistic science that fails to answer the most basic questions about consciousness or approach the enigma around the phenomena addressed through quantum physics (specifically the measurement problem).[10–12, 17–20]

The near-death experience community, as well as related spiritually-transformative experiences of all stripes, provides compelling evidence that consciousness is fundamental in the Universe. Spirituality and science strengthen each other greatly. Global awakening to this grand concept, not just among scientists but among all of us, is beginning even now.

CHAPTER TWELVE

Neuroscience Perspectives on Near-Death Experiences

Kevin Nelson, MD

Dr. Nelson explores near-death experiences through the lens of science and discovers that near-death fits within the conventional neuroscience framework as securely as the Germ Theory of Disease and Evolution stand in other branches of science.

In our time, near-death experiences (NDEs) dominate the discussion of spiritual experience. The drama of going through a tunnel, being enveloped by "the light," floating above one's body, and sometimes meeting deceased loved ones or spiritual beings constitutes a narrative thoroughly portrayed by the media. In the early twentieth century, American physician, philosopher and psychologist William James makes little mention of NDEs in his seminal work, *The Varieties of Religious Experience.* Yet, NDEs fulfills his expectation of a spiritual experience whereby "feelings, acts and experiences" touch "whatever they may consider the divine."[1]

Today's early twenty-first century view of these NDEs starts by first training our gaze on near-death's many overlooked scientific truths; some facts deliberately ignored and others simply neglected. So far, inundating the public with near-death topics has most served to reinforce media stereotypes rather than rooting out mistaken ideas.

"Near-Death" Is Often a Misnomer

For half of the instances of "near-death" the term is a misnomer because the person does not face imminent death. An excellent but seldom cited study examined the medical records of 58 people who experience near-death.[2]

Twenty-eight of those had a true medical crisis, while the other 30 were not medically endangered at the time. Surprisingly, the results showed almost identical experiences in both groups. Regardless of danger, people went through a tunnel, and had similar thoughts and emotions. Sixty-eight percent of all subjects had an out-of-body experience (OBE) whether they were medically near-death or not. The only physiologically interesting difference between their experiences intriguingly focused on "enhanced light" appearing to those truly endangered. These findings resonate with what else we know about the origins of near-death. Many things can cause NDEs including fear alone.[3, 4] Cardiac arrest stands among the most sensational triggers for NDEs, occurring in approximately 10% of survivors who recover with sufficient memory to recall the experience in some form.[5–7] (See Table 1.) Although this scenario features prominently in the public mind, it is not likely to top the list of causes for NDEs. We have yet to see a well-designed study in the general population, however, in a self-selected series of 55 subjects, syncope edged out cardiac events (10 versus 8).[8]

The role of syncope is crucial in NDEs. Syncope alone in the safely controlled environs of the neurophysiology laboratory produces features indistinguishable from NDE.[9, 10] This includes out-of-body experiences about 10% of the time. Upwards of one-third of people faint within their lifetime, often while feeling endangered, making syncope fertile ground for a spiritual experience. This may also explain why it was said that upwards of 18 million Americans may have had a near-death experience by a 1997 issue of *U.S. News & World Report.*

OUT-OF-BODY EXPERIENCE

Out-of-body experience (OBE), often a feature of near-death, is also an astoundingly frequent and normal experience separate from NDE. In a survey of over 13,000 individuals in the general population, 5.8% reported at least one OBE.[11] It is sobering to look upon a large crowd knowing that one in twenty have had an out-of-body experience. And like near-death, many physiologic factors lead to OBE. The common experience of syncope helps us understand the high incidence of OBE, but another physiologic state, a normal one, surely contributes as we shall soon see.

OBE accompanies near-death experiences 76% of the time.[12] Do OBE experiences always embody the qualities of spiritual experience? No! I have many subjects who regard their out-of-body experiences as a curiosity. One night drifting off to sleep, my psychiatric colleague floated a few feet above her bed and turned to see herself and husband beneath the quilt she crafted as a newlywed. She considered the intoxicating illusion "odd" but not profound. Many who have experienced OBE agree with the philosopher Descartes, not in his division of mind and brain, but when he said: "Whatever I have up till now accepted as most true I have acquired either from the senses or through the senses. But from time to time I have found that the senses deceive, and it is prudent never to trust completely those who have deceived us even once."[13] The OBE illusion is one of these sensory deceptions, and arises in the brain's temporoparietal region. Directly stimulating the temporoparietal cortex with a small electrical current evokes an OBE,[14,15] arguably by disturbing the integration of visual, proprioceptive and motion senses into the coherent self. In the laboratory or operating room, the neurophysiologist can bring a patient in and out of body, back and forth with the flip of a switch.

As important as NDEs have now become, another variety of spiritual experience reigns supreme by the fact that it is always and exclusively spiritual, and consequently the most historically influential variety serving as the "root and center" for organized religions of nearly every sort. James identified this experience as the "mystical sense of Oneness." Some of the many words use to describe the mystical Oneness include: boundless, ceaseless, bottomless, nothingness, fathomless, infinite, empty void, barren, abyss, abysmal, and absolute.

The philosopher W. T. Stace elaborated on the mystical nature brought out by James, noting that the core feeling of Oneness could be expressed in two forms.[16] The extrovertive mystical experience looks outward to the world through the physical senses and finds unity. On the other hand, the introvertive mystical experience turns inward, shuttering out the senses and transcending into a "pure" consciousness.

Both James and Stace believed the core nature of mystical experience was universal to humans. NDEs also appear universal but the narratives vary widely between persons and cultures, and are not always viewed in a spiritual perspective. Little thought has tied NDEs and mystical Oneness together until recently. A sizable 42 % of near-death experience subjects feel "united, one with the world."[8] Although not as thorough a measure as other tools provide, [17] this finding suggests that mystical Oneness may play an unsuspected role in making NDEs spiritual. This is important because much of the neuroscience behind mystical Oneness experience is understood.

MYSTICAL FEELINGS OF ONENESS

Mystical feelings of Oneness are expressed through a special quality of serotonin neurochemistry, specifically the serotonin-2a receptors. Much like a molecular scalpel, if serotonin-2a is pharmacologically blocked or parts of the limbic system containing serotonin-2a surgically removed, then the mystical expression is blocked too.

In retrospect the connection between NDE and the mystical Oneness should not come as a shock since fear, the primal emotion of the limbic system and survival, often accompanies mystical experiences. Which brings up another point; when exploring brain function during spiritually transforming experience it is not just the fervor over the drama of near-death that blinds some to the importance of the brain. The grandeur of the brain's accomplishments leads many to overlook the brain's prime biologic and evolutionary purpose lying at the heart of many spiritual experiences. First, last and, foremost the brain needs to keep itself alive through the crisis of near-death.

One extensively studied physiological crisis concerns cerebral blood flow. Crucial to its prime purpose, the brain governs its blood flow each second of life. Brain activity relies upon aerobic metabolism that demands a constant supply of oxygen and glucose at rest, in exercise, and during physiological and emotional stress. Controlling cerebral blood flow depends principally upon the arterial baroreflex that in turn pivots on the yoked opposition of cholinergic and adrenergic neurons in the peripheral and central nervous systems. Fading cerebral blood flow with looming unconsciousness, often the proximate circumstance leading to NDEs, signals a crisis to the brain that then orchestrates a cascade of survival responses, including the familiar fight-or-flight guiding our ancestors survival for millions of years. In the initial seconds of failing cerebral blood flow and dimming consciousness, there is no reason to expect the brain reacts differently between uncomplicated syncope and cardiac dysrhythmia.

When the brain becomes ischemic, many times the border between consciousness and unconsciousness is indistinct, and between these two borders exists a borderland of consciousness then entered. Consciousness is lost if blood flow drops below a threshold, and consciousness can come and go if cerebral blood flow rises and falls across this threshold; this routinely happens in clinical settings. It remains a scantly appreciated observation that the eyes remain open at syncope's onset[18] and beyond. So as consciousness waxes and wanes, a person may be far more aware of surrounding events than appreciated by others tending to medical urgencies. And those stricken may later recall the episode in startling detail. Simply because one does not respond while in shock or peri-syncopal does not mean the person is unconscious or dead (for example, see the case of Ms. Martin[19]). Adding to this caution, evidence suggests that the brain's electrical activity may persist even during deep coma and apparent isoelectric electroencephalogram.[20]

Although a misnomer a good part of the time, in one way the term "near-death experiences" aptly describes these experiences. They are not "return-from-death" experiences. Regrettably, some investigators use the term "clinical death" to "signify a period of unconsciousness caused by insufficient brain blood supply because of inadequate circulation, breathing, or both."[5] By this definition even harmless syncope is "clinical death" and we have already seen how this ambiguity can seriously mislead the unwary. Linking NDE to "clinical death" erroneously implies NDEs happen when the brain has died and the neurons lysed, a hallmark of neurologic brain death. Confusing cardiac dysrhythmia and "clinical death" has gone to extremes, leading one author to claim that these experiences are direct scientific evidence for "consciousness beyond life."[21]

One near-death experience has commanded so much media attention that it deserves some of ours, that of Eben Alexander III, MD, a neurosurgeon versed in neuroscience principles (see Chapter Eleven). In the midst of severe delirium from *E. coli* meningitis he describes a fantastic NDE sojourn. Later believing his brain had completely ceased functioning during his NDE, he titled his book, *Proof of Heaven*.[22] However, a simple question seemingly dismisses his contention: When in his delirium did the NDE arise? Since he provides no answer to that question, I believe there is no scientific basis to his assertion that his experience happened with his brain completely shut down.

Dr. Alexander's delirious memories do demonstrate one thing. The influence of a near-death experience can be powerful enough to conflate faith and science even in the mind of a neurosurgeon. They also show Descartes is once again correct, that our senses and the mental images derived from them can fool us about what we think we know.

The claims of Alexander, characterized by the eminent neurologist Oliver Sacks, MD, as anti-science, clash[23] with the sage words of a brilliant Canadian neurosurgeon from the mid-twentieth century. Wilder Penfield, MD, dedicated his career to electrically stimulating the brain, and his observations unveiled important new insights into the mysteries of mind and brain. He concluded that as scientists "we can only set out the data about the brain, and present the physiological hypotheses that are relevant to what the mind does." But as a human, he believed that "it is not unreasonable for him to *hope* [italics added] that after death the mind may waken to another source of energy."[24] Hope springs from faith, and there is room in the brain for faith.

A central tenet of neuroscience holds that all human experience arises from the brain,[25] akin to the Germ Theory of Disease and the Theory of Evolution in other branches of science. So far, the narratives of NDEs fit securely within the framework of conventional neuroscience. Sometimes I hear that neuroscience fails to explain a part of someone's recollection of their NDE; after allowing for selective, suggestible, reconstructed, and imperfect memory as well as the difficulty of knowing when in the crisis an experience occurred, nothing about NDEs, including OBEs, offers objective evidence that consciousness can exist without a living brain. Extraordinary claims require extraordinary evidence and here not even the most ordinary objective data supports the bold assertion of human consciousness outside the brain. When more facts become known in "unexplained" cases, a plausible neuroscience explanation has always been found. Belief in consciousness beyond the brain lies in the realm of faith beyond science. Faith has its place separate from science, in part because science has its limits imposed by the requirements of verification and reproducibility. Still, keep in mind that although not every scientific fact has been uncovered about black holes this still does not make black holes a supernatural force.

Alexander's book and others like *Heaven is Real* fall into a slick and clever literary genre of works taking the interpretation of near-death experiences as absolute and literal truth.[26] The literalist's success in the marketplace fails to substitute for evidence challenging the foundation of neuroscience.

Although science looks askance at the literalist take on NDEs, the literalists do raise a valid question. Do near-death experiences provide a glimpse of "The undiscover'd country, from whose bourn no traveller returns" (Hamlet, act 3, scene 1)? Of course we have no way of scientifically verifying if those having an NDE were on road, off road, made it part way, or almost all the way to that "undiscover'd country"(absolute death). The distance, direction, and destination of absolute death will never be proven scientifically.

Certainly if one posits the brain unnecessary for the sublime near-death experience, one can gloss over the arcane details of brain anatomy, chemistry, and physiology necessary to understand the brain's role. At the same time, for good reasons not everyone wants to know how the brain functions in spiritual experience. In an example from a different physiologic venue, I personally give little thought to my pancreatic juices as I dine on an excellent meal. My sister-in-law made clear to me why knowing how the brain works may not matter for a more important reason. Her father sustained a series of heart attacks and during one he left his body and calmly moved toward a warm glowing light. Afterwards he lost his fear of death and gained a new purpose in life, giving witness to the real, positive value of some NDEs. "I don't care what the brain is doing" she said, "I'm just happy with the comfort it gave dad."

But something deeper, something driving the neurologist within has set me on the quest for understanding NDEs. Split-brain studies from the 1970s unveiled the left cerebral hemisphere as the curious side, the one dominant for speech and symbolic understanding that also compels us to seek explanations for our experiences. There have been a host of offerings on what takes place in the brain during an NDE. Most flounder because of their simplicity by failing to recognize that the diversely rich experience of near-death surely draws upon more than a single physiological or biochemical system, or anatomical structure (See Table 1.).

Any neuroscience basis for NDEs must not only explain NDE features but provide a testable hypothesis and one that explains the relationship with syncope and the multitude of other triggers.

Many other factors must also be taken into account, factors that have received only the slightest attention. Since consciousness is central in many near-death

TABLE 1 Near-Death Features and Neuroscience Considerations Summarized

Near-Death Feature	Neuroscience Considerations
Tunnel	Retinal ischemia (common with systemic hypotension)
Light	Robust link with visual system (e.g., REM)
Appearing Dead	Atonia while alert
Out-of-body	Temporoparietal association
Life Review	Activating memory in the face of danger
Bliss	Dopamine reward system
Narrative Quality	Left hemisphere, limbic and other brain regions
Paranormal Impressions	Limbic system
Mystical Oneness	Serotonergic-2a receptors and limbic system

experiences, explanations must address mechanisms regulating consciousness. In crisis, survival demands an awake and attentive brain to meet the threat head on. This expectation seems so intuitively obvious that it typically escapes scrutiny. However, to survive the brain cannot take for granted being in the right conscious state at the right time. In waking consciousness attention suddenly orients to whatever survival requires. Therefore, consciousness and its altered states are bound to fight-or-flight action coordinated by the brainstem arousal and limbic systems. Essential to an effective survival response is the arousal system's locus coeruleus, the brain's nearly exclusive source of nor-epinephrine. The locus coeruleus is a minuscule cluster of pontine neurons key to regulating consciousness as well as survival behavior. This nucleus sends adrenergic neural projections throughout most of the entire brain.

RAPID EYE MOVEMENT CONSCIOUSNESS AND NDES

The strongest case for the neurophysiologic contribution to NDEs can be made for a borderland of consciousness. A borderland when the conscious states of waking and rapid eye movement (REM) blend, forming a hybrid conscious state. REM consciousness is named for the saccadic eye movements that accompany the robust visual system activation characterizing this conscious state. Cortical activation similar to wakefulness and the atonia of non-respiratory muscles also distinguish the REM state. The most complex dreaming takes place during REM sleep in cortical regions far removed from the pontine brainstem switch triggering REM. Importantly, these different elements of REM consciousness commonly fragment, and can individually intrude into the waking state. Most often the REM intrusion occurs in the transitions between REM and waking, happening in up to a quarter of people at least once in their life.[8] The blending of REM and waking consciousness takes the form of complex visual and auditory hallucinations, dream narratives, as well as the atonia of sleep paralysis or cataplexy. This borderland is unstable, lasting seconds or minutes before reverting to a more stable conscious state.

The REM intrusion hypothesis of near-death experiences was first investigated by discovering that those with a near-death experience have a 2.8 times greater incidence of lifetime REM intrusion than age and gender matched controls.[8] Near-death subjects possess a pontine REM switch so astoundingly predisposed to REM intrusion that the incidence of sleep paralysis does not differ between near-death and the sleep disorder of narcolepsy. Furthermore, for those who have been near death, REM intrusion happened with the same frequency before as after their near-death experience, telling us that near-death experience is but a single episode in a lifetime of REM intrusion.

To understand how conscious states interplay during a crisis like near-death, it is necessary to understand how the brainstem regulates consciousness and how the REM switch reacts in crisis to blend waking and REM consciousness bringing about effective survival behaviors. These details are beyond the scope of this review and chronicled more fully elsewhere.[27, 28] Table 2 summarizes the evidence that REM intrusion contributes to the near-death experience.

Another frequently overlooked fact is the long-established relationship between out-of-body and REM consciousness. Narcolepsy is a boundary of consciousness disorder whereby the afflicted suffer from REM frequently intruding into waking consciousness. Narcoleptics are very prone to out-of-body experience,[27, 29, 30] especially during sleep paralysis. The frequency of out-of-body wanes as the narcolepsy is treated. Out-of-body also appears in lucid dreams[31]—a special expression of dreaming wherein the dreamer maintains

TABLE 2 Summary of Evidence that REM Consciousness Contributes to Near Death*

Those with a near-death experience are strongly predisposed to life-long REM intrusion
Arousal electroencephalogram recorded after cardiac arrest
REM switch components linked to survival behavior that includes during systemic hypotension
Many clinical conditions provoke REM intrusion into waking consciousness
REM switch is part of the brainstem instrumental to the cardiovascular response to crisis (e.g., syncope/cardiac event)
Vagal nerve electrical stimulation briskly provokes REM intrusion
REM consciousness in situational context leads to many near-death features (e.g., out-of-body, paralysis, visual hallucinations, narrative, paralysis)

*A fuller discussion is found elsewhere.27, 28

insight while dreaming. In young healthy adults, OBE accompanies the sleep paralysis of REM intruding into waking consciousness.[32] (See Table 2.) The selective temporoparietal activity that normally takes place during REM[33] neatly explains the strong link between REM consciousness and OBEs. REM intrusion further explains the gripping feature of out-of-body often central to the NDE narrative and common in syncope. Further evidence of the bond between REM consciousness and NDEs comes from the observation that persons with a near-death experience are as likely to have OBE transitioning between waking and REM consciousness as they are to have it during NDE itself.[12] Their OBE often accompanies sleep paralysis.

Is REM intrusion the last word in NDE? Of course not! However, a notion sometimes expressed by those unfamiliar with the physiology of REM consciousness contends that near-death experiences do not engage REM mechanisms because NDE "doesn't feel like a dream." This assertion seems straightforward on the surface. After all, the memory of many near-death experiences that feels "realer than real" is at striking odds with the oftentimes outlandish, unreal, and faint impressions left by dreams upon awakening. Somehow this contention dismisses a crucial physiologic fact. Actually, we should expect different experiences from the same REM mechanism expressed under the very different conditions of routine sleep and an NDE. Context means much to experience. For example, temporoparietal brain stimulation in the laboratory evokes an OBE not unlike an OBE while piloting a fighter jet. So, too, the crisis of NDE brings its own context to influence an experience based upon the same brain physiologic mechanisms as REM sleep. One of my subjects, a severe narcoleptic with near daily REM intrusion, commonly has out-of-body experiences and nightly visions that feel every bit as real to him in the night as they do in the morning. Only through repeated occurrence does the true nature of REM intrusion reveal itself to him. He possesses no motivation, psychological or otherwise, to consider his illusions and hallucinations real. So the notion that NDEs are unrelated to REM because they do not feel like dreams carries little neuroscience weight. As a reminder, the feelings of deja vu caused by mesotemporal seizures leave an intensely real but false impression both during the seizure and afterwards.

In spite of the differences between near-death experiences and dream narratives, NDEs can be almost identical to lucid dreams, whereby the dreamer retains self-insight. This normal manifestation of dreaming conceivably arises when dorsolateral prefrontal cortical activity, instrumental to logical executive cognition and normally shut down during REM, persists during REM consciousness. Why some experiences seem real and others do not endures as a compelling question that applies to more experiences than just NDEs. Persisting dorsolateral prefrontal brain activity while REM blends with wakefulness in a moment when impaired cerebral metabolism struggles to sustain consciousness may deeply touch someone's impression of reality.

WHAT CAN WE CONCLUDE ABOUT NEAR-DEATH EXPERIENCES?

Clinicians must welcome near-death accounts with non-judgmental reassurance, providing safe harbor for patients with experiences that often bring overwhelming passions and memories. Medical professionals who tout spiritual shortcuts by forsaking science seriously risk debasing near-death experiences in the minds of many who hold science in esteem. We must not allow unsubstantiated literalists claims, playing upon popular sentiments, to tarnish the sincere near-death experience narrative.

In the end, the neuroscience of how the brain participates in near-death experiences does not demean their why or spiritual interpretation; these lie in the province of personal faith. Clinicians have an ethical responsibility to clearly differentiate the domains of science and faith, with respect to the power of near-death experiences to steadfastly transform personal meaning and spirituality. I urge heeding the advice of James when he drew upon biblical inspiration to counsel on spiritual experience: "by their fruits ye shall know them, not by their roots."[1]

CHAPTER THIRTEEN

Near-Death Experiences and the Emerging Scientific View of Consciousness

Eben Alexander III, MD

The phenomenological properties and transformative power of NDEs are totally different, and, in many ways, the opposite of dream content.

TOWARD A MORE COMPREHENSIVE SCIENTIFIC PARADIGM

I maintain that the human mystery is incredibly demeaned by scientific reductionism, with its claim in promissory materialism to account eventually for all of the spiritual world in terms of patterns of neuronal activity. This belief must be classed as a superstition . . . we have to recognize that we are spiritual beings with souls existing in a spiritual world as well as material beings with bodies and brains existing in a material world.

—Sir John C. Eccles, PhD, (1903–1997), neurophysiologist, Nobel Prize in Medicine and Physiology, 1963

ANY EVALUATION OF REPORTS OF near-death experiences must involve a mindset that is suitable to the task. These experiences challenge our understanding about the fundamental nature of consciousness, indeed of all of existence, at the most basic of levels, and if the mindset is too limited, we compromise our ability to approach the grander truth underlying our observations and attempts to understand them. The more broadly we can open our minds to the possibilities, the more readily we will come to a deeper understanding.

Kevin Nelson, MD's article in *Missouri Medicine*'s series on near-death experiences (NDEs) demonstrates the hazards of approaching near-death experiences with too limited a view of the possible explanations (Editor's note: Neuroscience Perspectives on Near-Death Experiences, 2015; 112 [2:92–98]). The danger lies in missing the forest for the trees, for being too myopic in scope and thus falling woefully short of the mark. This is an inherent problem when one is shackled, as is Dr. Nelson, within the narrow confines of the physicalist world view (i.e., that the physical world is all that exists; that consciousness is an epiphenomenon of the workings of the physical constituents of the brain following natural laws). By accepting the unproven assumption that the physical brain creates consciousness, his approach is doomed from the start. The brain is clearly related to consciousness—the fallacy is in believing the brain creates consciousness out of purely physical matter.

Entitled "Neuroscience Perspectives on Near-Death Experiences," Dr. Nelson's paper demonstrates many of the difficulties inherent in the scientific investigation of something as profoundly complex as near-death experiences when one's starting (physicalist) assumptions are false. The fog of confusion overwhelms his efforts to make sense of such deep experiences limited entirely to the confines of the physical brain, from a purely physicalist point of view.

In the teaser for his article, Dr. Nelson purports to "explore near-death experiences through the lens of science and discovers that near-death fits within the conventional neuroscience framework as securely as the Germ Theory of Disease and Evolution stand in other branches of science."

This teaser and his ensuing article address NDEs through a most distorted lens, indeed. First and foremost, Dr. Nelson seems to believe that conventional neuroscience has a firm enough understanding of the mechanism of consciousness to weigh in on all of the facets of near-death experiences. In fact, the "neuroscience of consciousness" is an oxymoron—no such entity exists. No neuroscientist on Earth, nor philosopher of mind, can offer even a few sentences in an effort to describe in broad strokes the mechanism by which the human brain might create consciousness—not even vague hand-waving. No one has a clue, and yet the mantra of conventional physicalist proponents like Nelson is that the brain creates consciousness, said with the conviction that it is such a well-established fact as to be beyond the necessity for any evidence.

Part of the unfathomable enigma of the relationship between brain and mind is reflected in what is known in scientific and philosophical circles as the "Hard Problem of Consciousness" (HPC), and many believe it is the most profound enigma in all of human thought. The HPC was defined by David Chalmers, PhD, as the challenge to physicalism in explaining "qualia," or the phenomenological aspects of human perceptions, and their integration into consciousness as a whole.[1] From a scientific perspective, it is challenging to even entertain possible questions that might lead toward experiments to better elucidate the mechanism of consciousness. The problem becomes less "hard" when one abandons the simplistic falsehoods of physicalism (i.e., that the brain creates consciousness). I believe that addressing the issue of consciousness more fully, as we do in this kind of discussion about near-death experiences, will lead us into fruitful territory in our understanding of the nature of reality and of humanity's place in it.

The conventional neuroscientific assertion that the brain creates the "illusion" of consciousness through the physical action of the subatomic particles, atoms, molecules, and cells of the brain, so fundamental to Dr. Nelson's point of view, is, as the Australian neurophysiologist and Nobel Laureate Sir John C. Eccles (quoted at beginning of article) famously said, "a superstition." Dr. Nelson and other physicalists are incapable of meeting the empirical challenges posed by the empirical data from NDEs, out-of body experiences (OBEs), and all manner of related mystical experiences. They neglect or deliberately ignore these "inconvenient" empirical facts, or attempt to explain away the basic rudiments through simplistic elementary explanations that cannot even begin to elucidate the rich landscape of the actual experiences.

As astrophysicist Paul Willard Merrill, PhD, wrote in his book on long-period variable stars, when faced with facts that contradict one's expectations, "if discordant values be omitted the others agree very well."[2] This humorous observation of science gone awry applies well to the approach of members of the conventional scientific community (like Nelson) who dismiss and deny any data from NDEs that do not fit rigidly into the conventional brain-creates-consciousness (physicalist) model.

A common error in this standard physicalist reasoning results from observing that some aspect x of NDEs (or OBEs) has some similarities to neurological condition y; therefore, explaining y explains those aspects x of NDEs, OBEs or other mystical experiences. This kind of oversimplification is guaranteed to lead to gross misinterpretation of the experiences.

Debunkers like Dr. Nelson don't acknowledge the differences between true OBEs and illusions of leaving the body. They then claim that explaining the illusions explains the real experiences. Most of the sources Nelson cites as explaining OBEs in fact explain a variety of somatic illusions that have nothing to do with OBEs, but are simply distortions of bodily perception that do not involve perception from an out-of-body perspective, to say nothing of cases of veridical perception from an out-of-body perspective.

"If all you have is a hammer, everything looks like a nail" also applies to modern neuroscience. Dr. Nelson has taken the physiology he feels he understands and applied it to these other phenomena, offering generic explanations based on weak analogies. One's tools and methodologies can confine one's ability to elucidate the underlying truth. It is better to stay focused on explaining the full experience as much as possible, remaining cognizant of the limitations of our tools and methodologies.

Nelson also ignores much of the relevant literature, including a voluminous amount of research on psi phenomena, the entire literature on survival of the soul after bodily death, the argument about deep general anesthesia presented in Irreducible Mind, the copious literature on cardiac arrest cases, and the transformative power of NDEs.[3] In addition, Nelson's discussion of OBEs focuses on illusory experiences, with no mention of the large literature on veridical OBEs.[4] The reasoning often implies that one non-veridical case means they all are.

In his discussion of how near-death is "often a misnomer," Dr. Nelson argues that in assessing the experiences in a mixed group of those who were medically near death and others who were not, that the experiences were quite similar between the two groups.[5] His interpretation misses the main point of that paper: the more dramatic changes in mentation occurred in patients who were medically closer to death, which directly confronts the notion that "brain creates mind." Nelson then tries to explain all NDEs as due to decreased cerebral blood flow. This shotgun approach is typical among the debunker/denier pseudo-skeptics—he can't have it both ways.

Nelson's claim that syncope produces features indistinguishable from an NDE reveals a fundamental misunderstanding of what an NDE actually is. I would compare this to claiming that the experience of viewing a partial eclipse of the sun is similar to that of viewing a total solar eclipse. Anyone who has witnessed the latter will understand what folly it is to assume that one can extrapolate the experience of a total eclipse from having viewed a partial eclipse.

Nelson's discussion of the mystical sense of Oneness (the "transcendent" aspect being the main contributor to an NDE's depth according to the Greyson scale) as being completely explicable through understanding the serotonin-2a receptor function in the brain is another example of how extreme oversimplification leads to erroneous conclusions. Correlation does not equal causality. If one is able to demonstrate changes in the brain through imaging with functional MRI, pharmacologic blockade, or similar means of evaluating brain function that occur during a specific phenomenal experience, that observation of putative correlation does not necessarily imply causality. Nelson's attempt to conflate fear and mystical experience is also erroneous and artificial.

Dr. Nelson claims that "much of the neuroscience behind mystical experience is understood"—a pretty bold claim, when in fact no neuroscientist on earth can offer even the most rudimentary statement about the neuroscience of consciousness, i.e., the mechanism by which the physical brain might give rise to consciousness.

THE INADEQUACY OF REM INTRUSION

Serious challenges to Dr. Nelson's proposed role of REM Intrusion in explaining the phenomena of NDEs have been pointed out by Bruce Greyson, MD, and Jeffrey P. Long, MD.[6]

Volunteers who share their NDEs on the internet, which comprise Nelson's study population, are probably more likely than most NDE experiencers in their willingness to publicly discuss unusual experiences

Nelson's control group, comprised of medical center personnel and their contacts, would have reservations about endorsing pathologic symptoms such as hallucinations, diminishing their value as a true control group (note their endorsement rate of only 7% for hypnagogic hallucinations, approximately one-fourth the rate in the general population).

Specific features such as fear, which is quite typical in sleep paralysis but rare in NDEs, as well as the occurrence of typical NDEs under general anesthesia and other drugs that inhibit REM, rule against any explanation of NDEs through REM intrusion.

The etiology of phenomena as complex as NDE is likely multi-factorial, making it unlikely that a single, simple physiologic explanation such as REM intrusion will suffice.

The phenomenological properties and transformative power of NDEs are totally different and, in many ways, the opposite of dream content. Spiritually transformative experiences of all sorts, including NDEs, are usually described as much more real than our daily reality in the physical realm. They are also life-altering, and much more persistent than the memories of dreams or hallucinations. To equate NDEs and dreams in the REM intrusion hypothesis is once again indicative of how one's prejudices and biases can lead one far astray.

PHYSICALISM IS INADEQUATE FOR THE TASK

In his comments about my coma experience,[7] Dr. Nelson incorrectly states that I "provided no answer to the question about when" in my coma the experience occurred. In fact, such an analysis was a crucial part of my investigation (as those who have actually read my book realize), and the clues within my odyssey revealed it all had to have occurred between days one and five of my seven-day coma, a period during which my neurologic examinations, imaging studies, and laboratory values all revealed my neocortex to be incapacitated by my meningitis.

Nelson concludes that "the influence of near-death experience can be powerful enough to conflate faith and science even in the mind of a neurosurgeon." In fact, the experience was powerful enough for this neurosurgeon to realize the brain does not create consciousness, to see the failure of pure physicalism as a worldview, to realize that mind or consciousness is primary (not brain or the physical realm), and to see the emergence of a natural synthesis of science and spirituality. It is our science that must expand its boundaries beyond the simplistic falsehoods of physicalism to more fully grasp the extreme mystery of consciousness as revealed through NDEs and similar experiences.

Nelson also claims this neurosurgeon to be "anti-scientific," then erroneously pits me against the "sage words of a brilliant Canadian neurosurgeon from the mid-twentieth century," Wilder Penfield, MD.[8] Dr. Nelson appears to have also completely misinterpreted Dr. Penfield's book and message, which, in fact, are closely aligned with my own view that the brain does not create the mind:

"But to expect the highest brain-mechanism or any set of reflexes, however complicated, to carry out what the mind does, and thus perform all the functions of the mind, is quite absurd." Penfield, p. 79

"And yet the mind seems to act independently of the brain in the same sense that a programmer acts independently of his computer, however much he may depend upon the action of that computer for certain purposes." Penfield, p. 79

"Taken either way, the nature of the mind presents the fundamental problem, perhaps the most difficult and most important of all problems. For myself, after a professional lifetime spent in trying to discover how the brain accounts for mind, it comes as a surprise now to discover, during this final examination of the evidence, that the dualist hypothesis seems the more reasonable of the two possible explanations." Penfield, p. 85 [i.e., that brain does not create mind, and the two should be considered as existing in their own right]

"What a thrill it is, then, to discover that the scientist, too, can legitimately believe in the existence of the spirit!" Penfield, p. 85

"The mind conditions the brain." Penfield, p. 86

"It is an observation relevant to any inquiry into the nature of man's being, and in conformity with the proposition that the mind has a separate existence. It might even be taken as an argument for the feasibility and the possibility of immortality!" Penfield, p. 87

"What is the reasonable hypothesis in regard to this matter, considering the physiological evidence? Only this: the brain has not explained mind fully." Penfield, p. 88

"I worked as a scientist trying to prove that the brain accounted for the mind and demonstrating as many brain-mechanisms as possible hoping to show how the brain did so. . . . In the end I conclude that there is no good evidence, in spite of new methods, such as the employment of stimulating electrodes, the study of conscious patients and the analysis of epileptic attacks that the brain alone can carry out the work that the mind does. I conclude that it is easier to rationalize man's being on the basis of two elements than on the basis of one." Penfield, pp. 113–114

Of note, Christof Koch, PhD, Chief Scientific Officer at the Allen Institute for Brain Science (Seattle), long a very determined physicalist neuroscientist, has recently followed Penfield in explicitly abandoning any hope of explaining consciousness as a product of brain processes. [9]

Nelson claims that "a central tenet of neuroscience holds that all human experience arises from the brain," which he erroneously concludes is aligned with the views of Penfield, whereas Penfield's (and my) position is exactly the opposite. Nelson claims that "a plausible neuroscience explanation has always been found in "unexplained" cases (especially of consciousness outside, or independent of, the brain)—another patently false assertion.

If one reads Dr. Penfield's book, and mine, they find we are congruent in many ways—certainly in stating that the brain does not create consciousness (the exact point Nelson is erroneously trying to contradict with his quote). Dr. Penfield's main limitations from that point, in my opinion, were not knowing enough about the implications of the measurement problem in quantum mechanics (not to mention the current experimental evidence supporting the "weirdness" of quantum reality, such as the recent "delayed choice quantum eraser" and related experiments[10, 11]), that it is information and not energy that is "conserved," and the fact that the current controversies in physics about the nature of causality that call into question our very notions of time itself[12, 13] had not yet emerged when Penfield wrote his insightful book in 1975.

Nelson demonstrates just how crippling blind faith in physicalism, the notion that "brain creates consciousness," can be. Others like him who widely trumpet this claim are guilty of an unsupported faith-based belief system, and of being willfully ignorant when they deny the data concerning the rich tapestry of mystical experiences, including NDEs.

In fact, the challenge of understanding NDEs from this brain-based perspective becomes even greater when one considers the realm of shared death experiences (SDEs), first described by Raymond Moody, MD, PhD, and Paul Perry in their fascinating book, *Glimpses of Eternity.*[14] The experiential aspects of SDEs closely resemble those of NDEs, but they occur in physiologically normal people. SDEs occur when the soul of a completely healthy bystander at the bedside of a dying patient is drawn along on the journey with the soul of the dying patient, even to the point of witnessing a full-blown life review of the departing soul, before the bystander soul returns to the earthly realm. In the hundreds of talks I give on these topics, I encounter numerous people who share their own stories of NDEs and after-death communications. A small but significant percentage of the stories I hear from the general public are actually of SDEs—they are not rare.

REJECTION OF THE DATA RESULTS IN WILLFUL IGNORANCE

Dr. Nelson is a neurologist who professes an interest in spiritual experiences. As such, one might expect him to demonstrate interest in the case of a neurosurgeon who was driven into coma over three hours due to gram-negative bacterial meningitis as severe as that which I reported in *Proof of Heaven,*[7] spent seven days in coma to the point where doctors had abandoned hope and were recommending termination of antibiotics, returned to this world with his mental faculties devastated, but then went on to a full recovery over eight weeks—to the point where he could participate in this deeply intellectual discussion about NDEs in *Missouri Medicine.* Yet Nelson's accusation that my book[7] "falls into a slick and clever literary genre," was based not on his having read the book, but on a book review article in the *New York Review of Books* by a literary critic (R Gottlieb) who was completely ignorant of the relevant scientific issues.[15] This reveals Nelson's unwillingness, or inability, to consider the relevant data, and to actually participate in this very deep discussion about the nature of consciousness and of all reality as revealed through NDEs and similar spiritually transformative experiences. Such willful ignorance is rampant among the debunkers and deniers of the physicalist camp, which renders their contribution to this deeper dialogue as largely irrelevant.

Nelson also does not appear to be familiar with the *Handbook of NDEs,*[4] *Irreducible Mind,*[3] or any other such books that responsibly address the full constellation of features found in NDEs, and in fact present a far more robust discussion of consciousness, and notably of non-local consciousness (i.e., consciousness independent of the here-and-now of the physical brain and body's immediate environs), than are found in any of the physicalist sources.

Part of the problem is that this is not simply a discussion about a few interesting and unusual phenomena that paradoxically appear around the time of death or near-death. Given that we are all essentially prisoners within our own consciousness, this discussion is actually about the very nature of all existence—a fundamental investigation into the nature of reality. A more comprehensive, top-down approach, one that takes all of the relevant data into account and addresses the profound mystery of our conscious existence itself might lead to a deeper understanding. Seeking answers is no small task: any significant progress will influence not only the realms of neuroscience and philosophy of mind, but the entire scientific community (notably physics and cosmology), and all of humanity.

SCIENCE BEYOND PHYSICALISM

If one is too confined by physicalist prejudices, e.g., believing at the outset that one is trying to fit the empirical observations into one's model of reality (i.e., that the brain creates the mind), they risk completely missing the deeper lessons of the journey. As with any attempt to gain a deeper understanding of something as fundamental as "consciousness," any partitioning of the subject matter is guaranteed to lead to confusion and misinterpretation. The problem is in our mindset, and is an inherent problem with the conventional scientific approach of reductive materialism.

The brain is clearly related to consciousness—the fallacy is in believing the brain creates consciousness out of purely physical matter. The emerging scientific view, far more powerful in its explanatory potential, relates to the notion of the brain as a reducing valve, or filter that limits primordial (infinite?) consciousness down to the minuscule trickle of the apparent here-and-now of our physical human existence. This idea (filter theory) enables the possibility that the soul survives bodily death, and is attributed to the brilliant masters of the human psyche who worked mainly in the late nineteenth and early twentieth centuries, notably Frederic W. H. Myers, Henri Bergson, and William James.[3]

Physicalism and atomism (the idea of the separation of objects within the universe) often go hand in hand—and both introduce distortions in trying to understand how humans fit into the universe as a whole. The act of separating parts of the universe from the whole is artificial and detracts from approaching the deeper truth of reality. This is one of the fundamental problems with our predominant scientific model of reductive materialism that relies largely on such false separations.

In spite of the wonders the world has seen from the advances of modern science and technology, there is a dark underbelly related to that progress in the form of the destruction of our planetary ecosystems, modern warfare, thoughtless homicide and suicide, etc.—much of it due to the artificial removal of human spirit from the predominant physicalist worldview.

The false conclusions of physicalist science that consciousness is manufactured by physiological processes occurring in the brain, that we are nothing more than "meat computers," automatons or zombies, that free will itself is a complete illusion, are vastly destructive as a predominant worldview. The emerging scientific view of consciousness as fundamental in the universe also incorporates the Oneness of all consciousness,[16] and the importance of appreciating the connectedness of all elements of the universe in reaching fundamental truth. I foresee this top-down approach to understanding as being much more fruitful.

For those with a serious interest in understanding the emerging science, I recommend especially the book *Beyond Physicalism: Toward Reconciliation of Science and Spirituality* (February 2015), edited by Edward F. Kelly, Adam Crabtree, and Paul Marshall, et. al from the Esalen Institute and the Division of Perceptual Studies at the University of Virginia. [17] This landmark opus, from the same group that published the world-changing *Irreducible Mind: Toward a Psychology for the 21st Century*,[3] offers a theoretical framework that will "hopefully contribute to blowing away the fog of ignorance and confusion that materialists have imposed on the scientific community and humanity at large," as stated by one of the prominent endorsers of the book, B. Alan Wallace, physicist, Buddhism scholar and teacher, and the president of the Santa Barbara Institute for Consciousness Studies. I agree wholeheartedly with Dr. Wallace's endorsement, which goes on to opine that *Beyond Physicalism* might allow us to "free ourselves from the ideological straitjacket of physicalism so that modern civilization can emerge from the dark age of ignorance and delusion about consciousness and return to the true spirit of open-minded empiricism that heralded the rise of modern science."

It is this open-minded empiricism to which I aspire, and which I encourage other scientific investigators to pursue. That is the spirit of this NDE series in *Missouri Medicine*—thus I felt compelled to respond to Dr. Nelson's article so that the physicalist/materialist camp was not claiming the final "scientific" word in this forum.

As much as Dr. Nelson claims to be holding up the light of science and reason, his physicalist view simply supports the "dark age of ignorance and delusion about consciousness," when true light and understanding are available—we must maintain an open mind and address all of the empirical data, not just that which we feel fits our dominant theoretical model. NDEs are just the tip of the iceberg in this evolving scientific view of the phenomena of non-local consciousness (proving the reality of phenomena such as near-death experiences, after-death communications, shared death experiences, telepathy, remote viewing, precognition, déjà vu, past-life memories in children indicative of reincarnation, psychokinesis, etc.).[3, 17]

A MASTERFUL ILLUSION

It is crucial to realize that the only thing any human being has ever experienced is the inside of his or her own consciousness, a model created within mind, but not external "objective" reality itself. Increasingly refined experiments in quantum mechanics suggest that there is no underlying objective reality—that all experience depends fundamentally on consciousness to allow its manifestation.[10, 11] There is no "clockwork universe" unfolding through pure natural laws, the object of natural science's attention during the Scientific Revolution (which began centuries ago, when scientists were less likely to tread on the sacred ground of mind and consciousness claimed by the powerful church, lest they be burned at the stake). All that is must be observed by mind in order to exist. As much as this defies our everyday assumptions, and the intentions of four centuries' of increasingly powerful probing by those pursuing investigations in the natural sciences, this is the way the universe works according to the most proven theory in the history of science (quantum mechanics). This is not some form of dogma, but in fact what is revealed in the most sophisticated efforts to probe the workings of the world, the very fabric of reality, at a subatomic level, through quantum physics.

The human brain and mind elaborate an astonishingly masterful illusion: every speck of our human experience and memory since before our birth has been our witnessing of an internal construct, of our mind's model of "reality," but not of reality itself. The profound consequences of this trick can lead us into a simplistic, unquestioning acceptance of the physicalist perspective, i.e., that only material stuff exists.

Given that our human perspective is always from within "mind," the greatest difficulty with assessing phenomena associated with near-death experiences is not having a broad enough field of view to get the full picture. The discussion rapidly converges around the fundamental nature of consciousness itself. This is the Mind-Body debate, an earnest and rigorous discussion that has been ongoing for ages, and formally for at least 2,600 years (since the likes of Plato, Aristotle, and Democritus weighed in with their often astonishingly prescient views). It is not surprising that more than a hundred generations of human beings have mused over the deep issues involved, but I find it astonishing that so little progress has been made. I also believe that this is about to change, and will involve a synthesis of the greatest wisdom from Eastern and Western spiritual traditions over millennia and the very frontiers of our current investigations in physics and cosmology.

In fact, the discussion goes far beyond the purview of just neuroscience and philosophy of mind—given that all of us are witnesses to our own mind only, it is about the fundamental nature of all reality and of our universe. All of physics and cosmology will participate in the emerging revelations from this discussion.

PONDERING THE UNKNOWN

> *Try and penetrate with our limited means the secrets of nature and you will find that, behind all the discernible concatenations, there remains something subtle, intangible and inexplicable. Veneration for this force beyond anything that we can comprehend is my religion. To that extent I am, in point of fact, religious.*
>
> —Albert Einstein (1879–1955)

The only safe assumption about the unknown is that it is infinite. Scientific inquiry over the last few centuries has proven that everyday human experience is often misleading in our effort to understand the true nature of reality. Proposing a "theory of everything" is a guaranteed source of embarrassment for the person foolish enough to believe they are close to such knowledge. Given that our modern society places scientists in such high esteem as the arbiters of truth, it is incumbent on scientists to fully admit the scope of the unknown in their endeavors.

The human pursuit of such deep understanding requires opening our minds broadly to explain all of our empirical observations. As Carl Sagan, PhD, so wisely pointed out, we are "not smart enough to know which pieces of knowledge are permissible"—thus scientists, first and foremost, should not suppress any knowledge, yet in the current discussion around NDEs the formal scientific community often actively denies and debunks everything that doesn't fit the very narrow physicalist model of "brain-creates-mind." Their unwarranted assumption that the brain creates consciousness renders their contribution to any meaningful discussion of NDEs as woefully impotent.

Much of our knowledge about the nature of reality must derive from all of human experience, not just the limited flow from strict application of the scientific method in a controlled environment. Anecdotes provide a rich source of understanding, if they are carefully scrutinized and combined with other knowledge. In fact, all of scientific discovery has involved anecdotes and individual experience as the seed from which knowledge emerges.

The good news is that many scientists around the world fully appreciate the depth of the mystery of consciousness, and how NDEs and similar mystical experiences offer profound clues in approaching a deeper understanding of the underlying reality.[18] This dialog sows the seeds for the destruction of the purely physicalist model of the universe. Likewise, the startling enigma of the measurement problem in quantum mechanics, which suggests that consciousness is primordial in the universe, calls for a fundamental reworking of our worldview.[10] Current scientific understanding must be greatly expanded to fully incorporate the unfathomably deep mystery of consciousness itself and its role in manifesting all of emergent reality.

Nelson closes his article with: "Medical professionals who tout spiritual shortcuts by forsaking science seriously risk debasing near-death experiences in the minds of many who hold science in esteem. . . . Clinicians have an ethical responsibility to clearly differentiate the domains of science and faith."

In fact, Nelson is the one guilty of "forsaking science." The emerging scientific view will be one that fully embraces these extraordinary conscious experiences and provides a far more realistic model of the universe than the paltry and barren fiction provided by lame physicalism.

I believe that medical professionals like Nelson who claim to have purely materialist explanations of phenomena that are far beyond the ken of those simplistic "scientific" physicalist assumptions do great damage in pretending they know things they do not, such as the mechanism of consciousness itself—therein lies the real damage that can be done in the interaction between medical professionals and their patients who report these amazing journeys.

We ought rather to foster an environment where these stories are widely shared and discussed—they are gems that reward us with great riches in a deeper understanding of all of existence. The expanding boundaries of this emerging science will fully embrace our spirituality and allow medical professionals who are more enlightened to offer greater healing than the purely physicalist mindset ever allowed.

Contributors

Eben Alexander III, MD, is a former neurosurgeon who spent fifteen years on faculty at Harvard Medical School, the Brigham & Women's and the Children's Hospitals in Boston, MA. He wrote a memoir about his near-death experience entitled *Proof of Heaven: A Neurosurgeon's Journey into the Afterlife* (2012), and has written a comprehensive sequel entitled *The Map of Heaven: How Science, Religion and Ordinary People are Proving the Afterlife* (2014). Contact: ealexanderiii@earthlink.net.

Nancy Evans Bush, MA, is President Emerita, International Association for Near-Death Studies. Contact: nanbush5@gmail.com.

Tony Cicoria, MD, is an orthopedic surgeon, and chief of orthopedics at Chenango Memorial Hospital, Norwich, New York, and Clinical Assistant Professor of Orthopedics at SUNY Upstate Medical School, in Syracuse. Jordan Cicoria, Dr. Cicoria's daughter, is a recent graduate of the University of Rochester, and a writer, and plans to attend graduate school. Contact: tcicoria @gmail.com.

Bruce Greyson, MD, is the Chester F. Carlson Professor of Psychiatry and Neurobehavioral Sciences and former Director of the Division of Perceptual Studies at the University of Virginia School of Medicine. Contact: cbg4d @virginia.edu.

John C. Hagan III, MD, is a Fellow of the American College of Surgeons and the American Academy of Ophthalmology. A prolific clinical researcher, he has published over 180 papers in peer-reviewed journals and co-edited the text *Care of the Dying Patient* (Missouri University Press, 2010). He is an award-winning writer and has served as editor of *Missouri Medicine* since 2000. He is listed in *American's Best Ophthalmologists* and serves in leadership of numerous state and national professional organizations. Contact: jhagan @bizkc.rr.com.

Jean Renee Hausheer, MD, FACS, was an MSMA member from 1986 to 2011 and served twice on the Missouri Board of Healing Arts. She moved to Oklahoma in 2011 where she is Clinical Professor of Ophthalmology, Dean McGee Eye Institute, University of Oklahoma School of Medicine. She practices in Lawton, Oklahoma. Contact: dr.jean.hausheer@gmail.com.

Janice Miner Holden, EdD, is Chair, Department of Counseling and Higher Education and Professor, Counseling Program, College of Education, University of North Texas. She is the editor of the *Journal of Near-Death Studies* and Past-President of The International Association for Near-Death Studies (IANDS). Contact: Jan.Holden@unt.edu.

Pim van Lommel, MD, worked from 1977 to 2003 as a cardiologist in Hospital Rijnstate, a teaching hospital in Arnhem, the Netherlands, and is now doing full-time research on the mind-brain relationship. Through his research on near-death experiences in survivors of cardiac arrest, he is the author of over thirty articles, one book, and several chapters about NDE. Contact: pimvanlommel@gmail.com.

Jeffrey Long, MD, is a radiation oncologist in Houma, Louisiana, and a recognized world expert on near-death experiences. Dr. Long established the nonprofit Near Death Experience Research Foundation and a website forum (www.nderf.org) for people to share their NDEs. Contact: nderf@nderf.org.

Raymond Moody, MD, PhD, is a world-renowned author, lecturer, and psychiatrist whose seminal book, *Life After Life*, completely changed the way death and dying are viewed. He is widely acknowledged as the world's leading expert in the field of near-death studies. His books are perennial best sellers and over 20 million have been sold. Contact: Raymond@LifeAfterLife.com.

Kevin Nelson, MD, is Professor of Neurology at the University of Kentucky engaged in the clinical practice of neurophysiology for thirty years, as well as Director of Medical Affairs for nearly twenty years. He is author of the book *The Spiritual Doorway in the Brain*. Contact: knelson@uky.edu.

Dean Radin, PhD, is Chief Scientist at the Institute of Noetic Sciences (IONS) and Adjunct Faculty in the Department of Psychology at Sonoma State University. He is former President of the Parapsychological Association and co-editor-in-chief of the journal *Explore: The Journal of Science and Healing*. Contact: dradin@noetic.org.

Penny Sartori, RN, PhD, has worked as an intensive care nurse for over two decades. She conducted the first prospective long-term study on near-death experiences in the United Kingdom. She has special expertise and interest in NDEs in children and has published and lectures extensively on the subject. Contact: p.sartori@ntlworld.com.

Notes

Chapter One: Near-Death Experiences: An Essay in Medicine & Philosophy
Originally published September/October 2013, *Missouri Medicine, 110*, 5.

1. Moody, R. A., Jr. (2001). *Life after life: The 25th anniversary of the classic bestseller.* San Francisco, CA: HarperOne.

2. Moody, R. A., Jr. (1975). *Life after life: The investigation of a phenomenon—survival of bodily death.* New York, NY: MMB, Inc. (later Bantam Books). http://www. lifeafterlife.com

3. Guthrie, W. K. C. (1979). *A history of Greek philosophy: Volume 2, The presocratic tradition from Parmenides to Democritus.* Cambridge, UK: Cambridge University Press: 436–438.

4. Plato. (circa 380 BC). *The Republic.*

Chapter Two: An Overview of Near-Death Experiences
Originally published November/December 2013, *Missouri Medicine, 110*, 6.

1. Noyes, R., & Kletti, R. (1972). The experience of dying from falls. *Omega, 3*, 45–52.

2. Moody, R. A., Jr. (1975). *Life after life: The investigation of a phenomenon—survival of bodily death.* New York, NY: MMB, Inc. (later Bantam Books). http://www.lifeafterlife.com

3. Zingrone, N. L., & Alvarado, C. S. (2009). Pleasurable Western adult near-death experiences: Features, circumstances, and incidence. In J. M. Holden, B. Greyson, & D. James (Eds.), *The handbook of near-death experiences: Thirty years of investigation.* Santa Barbara, CA: Praeger/ABC-CLIO: 17–40.

4. Van Lommel, P. (2011). Near-death experiences: The experience of the self as real and not as an illusion. *Annals of the New York Academy of the Sciences, 1234*, 19–28.

5. Holden, J. M., Greyson, B., & James, D. (Eds). (2009). *The handbook of near-death experiences: Thirty years of investigation.* Santa Barbara, CA: Praeger/ABC-CLIO.

6. Noyes, R., Fenwick, P., Holden, J. M., & Christian, S. R. (2009). Aftereffects of pleasurable Western adult near-death experiences. In J. M. Holden, B. Greyson, & D.

James (Eds.), *The handbook of near-death experiences: Thirty years of investigation.* Santa Barbara, CA: Praeger/ABC-CLIO: 41–62.

7. Greyson, B. (2007). Near-death experiences: Clinical implications. *Revista de Psiquiatria Clínica, 34*(Suppl. 1), 49–57.

8. Parnia, S., & Fenwick, P. (2002). Near death experiences in cardiac arrest: Visions of a dying brain or visions of a new science of consciousness? *Resuscitation, 52,* 5–11.

9. Thonnard, M., Charland-Verville, V., Bredart, S., Dehon, H., Ledoux, D., Laureys, S., & Vanhaudenhuyse, A. (2013). Characteristics of near-death experiences memories as compared to real and imagined events memories. *PLoS ONE, 8*(3): e57620.

10. Greyson, B. (2007). Consistency of near-death experience accounts over two decades: Are reports embellished over time? *Resuscitation, 73,* 407–411.

11. Holden, J. M., Long, J., & MacLurg, B. J. (2009). Characteristics of western near-death experiencers. In J. M. Holden, B. Greyson, & D. James (Eds.), *The handbook of near-death experiences: Thirty years of investigation.* Santa Barbara, CA: Praeger/ABC-CLIO 2009: 109–133.

12. Athappilly, G. K., Greyson, B, & Stevenson, I. (2006). Do prevailing societal models influence reports of near-death experiences? *Journal of Nervous & Mental Disease, 194,* 218–222.

13. Kellehear, A. (2009). Census of non-western near-death experiences to 2005. In J. M. Holden, B. Greyson, & D. James (Eds.), *The handbook of near-death experiences: Thirty years of investigation.* Santa Barbara, CA: Praeger/ABC-CLIO: 135–158.

14. Greyson, B., Kelly E. W., & Kelly E. F. (2009). Explanatory models for near-death experiences. In J. M. Holden, B. Greyson, & D. James (Eds.), *The handbook of near-death experiences: Thirty years of investigation.* Santa Barbara, CA: Praeger/ABC-CLIO: 213–234.

15. Greyson, B. (2013). Near-death experiences. In E. Cardeña, S. J. Lynn, S. Krippner (Eds.), *Varieties of anomalous experience: Examining the scientific evidence* (2nd ed.). Washington, DC: American Psychological Association: 333–367.

16. Britton, W. B., Bootzin, R. R. (2004). Near-death experiences and the temporal lobe. *Psychological Science, 15,* 254–258.

17. Kelly, E. W., Greyson, B., & Kelly, E. F. (2006). Unusual experiences near death and related phenomena. In E. F. Kelly, E. W. Kelly, A. Crabtree, A. Gauld, M. Grosso, & B. Greyson (Eds.), Irreducible mind: Toward a psychology for the 21st century. Lanham, MD: Rowman & Littlefield: 367–421.

18. Greyson, B. (1997). The near-death experience as a focus of clinical attention. *Journal of Nervous & Mental Disease,185,* 327–334.

19. Bush, N. E. (1991). Is ten years a life review? *Journal of Near-Death Studies, 10,* 5–9.

20. Greyson, B. (2003). Near-death experiences in a psychiatric outpatient clinic population. *Psychiatric Services, 54,* 1649–1651.

21. Holden, J. M. (2009). Veridical perception in near-death experiences. In J. M. Holden, B. Greyson, & D. James (Eds.), *The handbook of near-death experiences: Thirty years of investigation.* Santa Barbara, CA: Praeger/ABC-CLIO: 185–211.

22. Greyson, B. (2010). Implications of near-death experiences for a postmaterialist psychology. *Psychology of Religion and Spirituality, 2,* 37–45.

23. Greyson, B. (2010). Seeing dead people not known to have died. *Anthropology & Humanism, 35,* 159–171.

24. Facco, E., & Agrillo, C. (2012). Near-death experiences between science and prejudice. *Frontiers in Human Neuroscience, 6,* 209. doi: 10. 3389/fnhum. 2012. 00209

Chapter Three: Out of One's Mind or Beyond the Brain?
The Challenge of Interpreting Near-Death Experiences

Originally published January/February 2014, *Missouri Medicine, 111,* 1.

1. Crick, F. (1994). *The astonishing hypothesis: The scientific search for the soul.* New York, NY: Touchstone.

2. McNamara, J. (2012). Brain Facts: A primer on the brain and nervous system In *Society for Neuroscience* (Ed.), (7 ed.). Washington, DC: Society for Neuroscience.

3. Van Lommel, P. (2010). *Consciousness beyond life: The science of the near-death experience.* San Francisco, CA: HarperOne.

4. Van Lommel, P., Van Wees, R., Meyers, V., & Elfferich, I. (2001). *Lancet, 358*(9298), 2039–2045.

5. Kroeger, D., Florea, B., & Amzica, F. (2013). *PloS ONE, 8*(9), e75257.

6. Borjigin, J., Lee, U., Liu, T., Pal, D., Huff, S., Klarr, D., Sloboda, J., Hernandez, J., Wang, M. M., & Mashour, G. A. (2013). *PNAS, 110,* 14432–14437.

7. Greyson, B. (2007). *Resuscitation, 73*(3), 407–411.

8. Radin, D. I. (1997). *The conscious universe: the scientific truth of psychic phenomena.* New York, NY: HarperEdge.

9. Radin, D. I. (2006). *Entangled minds: Extrasensory experiences in a quantum reality.* New York, NY: Paraview Pocket Books.

10. Rhine, J. B. (1934). *Extra-sensory perception.* Boston, MA: Boston Society for Psychic Research.

11. Pratt, J. G., Rhine, J. B., Smith, B. M., Stuart, C. E., & Greenwood, J. A. (1940). *Extra-sensory perception after sixty years: A critical appraisal of the research in extra-sensory perception.* New York, NY: H. Holt and Company.

12. Teuscher, C. (2004). *Alan Turing: Life and legacy of a great thinker.* New York, NY/Berlin, Germany: Springer.

13. Turing, A. M. (1950). *Mind, 59,* 433–460.

14. Skinner, B. F. (1976). *About behaviorism.* New York, NY: Vintage Books.

15. Penman, D. (2008) *The Daily Mail* http://www.dailymail.co.uk/news/article-510762/could-proof-theory-ALL-psychic.html (accessed 16 Feb. 2010).

16. Radin, D. I. (2013). *Supernormal: Science, yoga, and the evidence for extraordinary psychic abilities.* New York, NY: Random House.

17. Tressoldi, P. E., Storm L., & Radin, D. (2010). *NeuroQuantology, 8*(4, Suppl.1), S81–87.

18. Delgado-Romero, E. A., & Howard, G. S. (2005). *The Humanistic Psychologist, 33*(4), 293–303.

19. Tressoldi, P. E. (2011). *Frontiers in Psychology, 2.*

20. Schmidt, S., Scheider, R., Utts, J., & Walach, H. (2004). *British Journal of Psychology, 95,* 235.

21. Duane, T. D., & Behrendt, T. (1965). *Science, 150,* 367.

22. Targ, R., & Puthoff, H. (1974). *Nature, 252,* 602–607.

23. Radin, D. I. (2004). *Journal of Alternative and Complementary Medicine, 10,* 315–324.

24. Standish, L. J., Kozak, L. Johnson, L. C., & Richards, T. (2004). *Journal of Alternative and Complementary Medicine, 10,* 307–314.

25. Wackermann, J., Seiter, C., Keibel, H., & Walach, H. (2003). *Neuroscience Letters, 336,* 60–64.

26. Standish, L. J., Johnson, L., Kozak C. L., & Richards, T. (2003). *Alternative Therapies, 9,* 122–125.

27. Richards, L., Kozak, T. L., Johnson L. C., & Standish, L. J. (2005). *Journal of Alternative and Complementary Medicine, 11*(6), 955–963.

28. Achterberg, J., Cooke, K., Richards, T., Standish L. J., & Kozak, L. (2005). *Journal of Alternative and Complementary Medicine,* 11(6), 965–971.

29. Dunne, B. J., & Jahn, R. G. (2007). *Explore* (NY), *3*(3), 254–269, 343–254.

30. Mossbridge, J., Tressoldi, P., & Utts, J. (2012). *Frontiers in Perception Science, 3,* 1–18.

31. Bem, D. J. (2011). *Journal of Personality and Social Psychology, 100*(3), 407–425.

32. Radin, D.I., Michel, L., Galdamez, K., Wendland, P., Rickenbach, R., & Delorme, A. (2012). *Physics Essays, 25*(2), 157–171.

33. Radin, D., & Nelson, R. (1989). *Found Physics, 19,* 1499.

34. Vane, J. R., & Botting, R. M. (2003). *Thrombosis Research, 110,* 255–258.

35. Verschuur, G. L. (1993). *Hidden attraction: The history and mystery of magnetism.* Oxford, UK: Oxford University Press.

36. Chalmers, D. J. (2010). *The character of consciousness.* New York, NY: Oxford University Press, USA.

37. Searle, J. R., Dennett, D. C., & Chalmers, D. J. (1997). *The mystery of consciousness.* New York, NY: New York Review of Books.

38. Beischel, J., & Schwartz, G. E. (2007). *Explore* (NY), *3*(1), 23–27.

39. Beischel, J. (2011). *Journal of Nervous and Mental Disease, 199*(6), 425–426; author reply 426.

Chapter Four: Dutch Prospective Research on Near-Death Experiences during Cardiac Arrest

Originally published March/April 2014, *Missouri Medicine, 111,* 2.

1. Van Lommel, P. (2010). *Consciousness beyond life: The science of the near-death experience* (L. Vroomen, Trans.). New York, NY: HarperCollins. (Originally published as *Eindeloos bewustzijn: Een wetenschappelijke visie op de bijna-dood ervaring* in 2007 by Kampen, The Netherlands: Ten Have Publishing)

2. Gallup, G., & Proctor, W. (1982). *Adventures in immortality: A look beyond the threshold of death.* New York, NY: McGraw-Hill.

3. Schmied, I., Knoblaub, H., & Schnettler, B. (1999). *Todesnäheerfahrungen in Ost- und Westdeutschland: Eine empirische Untersuchung.* In H. Knoblaub & H. G. Soeffner (Eds.), *Todesnähe: Interdisziplinäre Zugänge zu Einem Außergewöhnlichen Phänomen.* Konstanz, Germany: Universitätsverlag Konstanz: 65–99.

4. Van Lommel, P., van Wees, R., Meyers, V., & Elfferich, I. (2001). Near-death experiences in survivors of cardiac arrest: A prospective study in the Netherlands. *Lancet, 358,* 2039–2045.

5. Ring, K. (1980). *Life at death: A scientific investigation of the near-death experience.* New York, NY: Coward, McCann & Geoghegan.

6. Van Lommel, P. (2010). *Consciousness beyond life: The science of the near-death experience* (L. Vroomen, Trans.). New York, NY: HarperCollins. (Originally published as *Eindeloos bewustzijn: Een wetenschappelijke visie op de bijna-dood ervaring* in 2007 by Kampen, The Netherlands: Ten Have Publishing)

7. Greyson, B. (2003). Incidence and correlates of near-death experiences in a cardiac care unit. *General Hospital Psychiatry, 25,* 269–276.

8. Parnia, S., Waller, D. G., Yeates, R., & Fenwick, P. A. (2001). A qualitative and quantitative study of the incidence, features and aetiology of near death experience in cardiac arrest survivors. *Resuscitation, 48,* 149–156.

9. Sartori, P. (2006). The incidence and phenomenology of near-death experiences. *Network Review* (Scientific and Medical Network), *90,* 23–25.

10. Van Lommel, P. (2013). Non-local consciousness: A concept based on scientific research on near-death experiences during cardiac arrest. *Journal of Consciousness Studies, 20*(1–2), 7–48.

11. Ring, K., & Cooper, S. (1999). *Mindsight: Near-death and out-of-body experiences in the blind.* Palo Alto, CA: William James Center for Consciousness Studies.

12. Van Lommel, P. (2010). *Consciousness beyond life: The science of the near-death experience* (L. Vroomen, Trans.). New York, NY: HarperCollins. (Originally published as *Eindeloos bewustzijn: Een wetenschappelijke visie op de bijna-dood ervaring* in 2007 by Kampen, The Netherlands: Ten Have Publishing)

13. Van Lommel, P. (2013). Non-local consciousness: A concept based on scientific research on near-death experiences during cardiac arrest. *Journal of Consciousness Studies, 20* (1–2), 7–48.

14. Benedetti, F., Mayberg, H. S., Wager, T. D., Stohler, C. S., & Zubieta, J. K. (2005). Neurobiological mechanisms of the placebo effect. *Journal of Neuroscience,* 25(45), 10390–10402.

15. Beauregard, M. (2007). Mind does really matter: Evidence from neuroimaging studies of emotional self-regulation, psychotherapy, and placebo effect. *Progress in Neurobiology, 81*(4), 218–236.

Chapter Five: My Unimaginable Journey: A Physician's Near-Death Experience

Originally published May/June 2014, *Missouri Medicine*; *111*, 3.

Chapter Six: My Near-Death Experience: A Call from God

Originally published July/August 2014, *Missouri Medicine*, *111*, 4.

1. Sacks, O. (2007). *Musicophilia: Tales of music and the brain.* New York, NY: Knopf.

2. Sacks, O. (2012). *Hallucinations.* New York, NY: Knopf.

3. Treffert, D. (2010). *Islands of genius: The bountiful mind of the autistic, acquired, and sudden savant.* London, UK: Jessica Kingsley.

4. PBS-WSKG. (2008). Tony Cicoria [Television series episode]. In *Expressions: The Art and Soul of the Southern Tier.* WSKG-PBS-NPR Production.

5. PBS-NOVA. (2009). Musical Minds with Dr. Oliver Sacks. Can the Power of Music Make the Brain Come Alive? [Television series episode]. In *Nova*. BBC Production; PBS-NOVA. (2009). The Music Instinct: Science and Song. [Television series episode]. In *Nova*. Elena Mannes Production.

6. Moody, R. A., Jr. (1975). *Life after life.* Covington, GA: Mockingbird Books.

7. Sacks, O. W. (2012, December 12). Seeing God in the third millennium: How the brain creates out of body experiences and religious epiphanies. *The Atlantic.*

8. Sabom, M. (1998). *Light and death: One doctor's fascinating account of near-death experiences.* Grand Rapids, MI: Zondervan Publishing House.

9. Holden, J. Personal communication (2013, 2014).

10. Woerlee, G. (2011). Could Pam Reynolds hear? A new investigation into the probability of hearing during this famous near death experience. *Journal of Near Death Studies*, *30*(1), 3–25.

11. Van Lommel, P., van Weis, R., Meyers, V., & Elfferich, I. (2001). Near-death experience in survivors of cardiac arrest: A prospective study in the Netherlands. *Lancet*, *58*, 2039–2045.

12. Van Lommel, P. (2010) *Consciousness beyond life: The science of the near-death experience* (L. Vroomen, Trans.). New York, NY: HarperCollins. (Originally published as *Eindeloos bewustzijn: Een wetenschappelijke visie op de bijna-dood ervaring* in 2007 by Kampen, The Netherlands: Ten Have Publishing)

13. Van Lommel, P. (2011). Near-death experiences: The experience of the self as real and not as an illusion. *ANYAS*, *1234*, 19–28.

14. Parnia, S., Waller, D., Yeates, R., & Fenwick, P. (2001). A qualitative and quantitative study of the incidence, features, and aetiology of near-death experiences in cardiac arrest survivors. *Resuscitation*, *48*(2), 149–156.

15. Morse, M. (1996). *Parting visions: A new scientific paradigm.* In L. W. Baily & J. Yates (Eds.), *The near-death experience: A reader.* New York, NY/London, UK: Routledge: 299–318.

16. Ring, K., & Cooper, S. (1999). *Mindsight: Near-death and out-of-body experiences in the blind.* Palo Alto, CA: William James Center for Consciousness Studies.

17. Penfield, W. (1955). "The role of the temporal cortex in certain psychical phenomena. *Journal of Mental Science*, *101*, 451–465.

18. Penfield, W. (1958). *The excitable cortex in conscious man.* Liverpool, UK: Liverpool University Press.

19. Blanke, O., Landis, T., Spinelli, L., & Seeck, M. (2004). Out of body experience and autoscopy of neurological origin. *Brain, 127*(2), 243–258.

20. Nelson, K., Mattingly, M., Lee, S., & Schmitt, F. (2006). Does the arousal system contribute to near-death experiences? *Neurology, 66*, 1003–1009.

21. Nelson, K., Mattingly, M., & Schmitt, F. (2007). Out of body experience and arousal. *Neurology, 68*, 794–795.

22. Borjigin, J., et al. (2013). Surge of neurophysiological coherence and connectivity in the dying brain. *PNAS, 110*(35), 14432–14437.

23. Chawla, L, Akst, S., Junker, C., Jacobs, B, Seneff, M. "Surges of EEG activity at the time of death: a case series." J. Palliative Med. 2009; 12(12): 1095–1100.

24. Brinkley, D., Perry, P., & Moody, R. (1995) *Saved by the light.* New York, NY: HarperOne.

25. Burpo, T., & Vincent, L. (2010). *Heaven is for real.* Nashville, TN: Thomas Nelson.

26. Plato. (circa 380 BC). *The Republic.*

27. Pythagoras. Are numbers gods? In C. Pickover (2009), *The loom of God: Tapestries of mathematics and mysticism.* New York, NY/London, UK: Sterling Publishing: 35.

28. Holden, J. M., Greyson, B., & James, D. (Eds). (2009). *The handbook of near-death experiences: Thirty years of investigation.* Santa Barbara, CA: Praeger/ABC-CLIO.

29. Morse, M., & Perry, P. (2000). *Where God lives: The science of the paranormal and how our brains are linked to the universe.* San Francisco, CA: Harper San Francisco.

30. Kelly, R. (2007). *The Human Antenna.* Santa Barbara, CA: Energy Psychology Press.

Chapter Seven: Near-Death Experiences: Evidence for Their Reality

Originally published September/October 2014, *Missouri Medicine, 111*, 5.

1. Zingrone, N. L., & Alvarado, C. S. (2009). Pleasurable Western adult near-death experiences: Features, circumstances, and incidence. In J. M. Holden, B. Greyson, & D. James (Eds.), *The handbook of near-death experiences: Thirty years of investigation.* Santa Barbara, CA: Praeger/ABC-CLIO:17–40.

2. Moody, R. A., Jr. (1975). *Life after life.* Covington, GA: Mockingbird Books.

3. Greyson, B. (2003). The Near-death experience scale: Construction, reliability and validity. *Journal of Nervous and Mental Disease, 171*, 369–375.

4. http://www.nderf.org/NDERF/EvidenceAfterlife/Survey_Internet_Pencil_Paper.htm

5. Sabom, M. (1982). *Recollections of death: A medical investigation.* New York, NY: Simon & Schuster; Van Lommel, P., van Wees, R., Meyers, V., & Elfferich, I. (2001). Near-death experience in survivors of cardiac arrest: A prospective study in the Netherlands. *Lancet, 358*, 2039–45; Parnia, S., Waller, D. G., Yeates, R., & Fenwick, P. (2001). A qualitative and quantitative study of the incidence, features and aetiology of near death experiences in cardiac arrest survivors. *Resuscitation*, 48, 149–156; Schwaninger, J., Eisenberg, P. R., Schechtman, K. B., & Weiss, A. N. (2002). A prospective analysis

of near-death experiences in cardiac arrest patients. *Journal of Near-Death Studies, 20,* 215–232; Greyson, B. (2003). Incidence and correlates of near-death experiences in a cardiac care unit. *General Hospital Psychiatry, 25,* 269–276.

6. DeVries, J. W., Bakker, P. F. A., Visser, G. H, Diephuis, J. C., & van Huffelen, A. C. (1998). Changes in cerebral oxygen uptake and cerebral electrical activity during defibrillation threshold testing. *Anesthesiology and Analgesia, 87,* 16–20.

7. Aminoff, M. J., Scheinman, M. M., Griffin, J. C., & Herre, J. M. (1988). Electrocerebral accompaniments of syncope associated with malignant ventricular arrhythmias. *Annals of Internal Medicine, 108,* 791–796; Van Lommel, P., van Wees, R., Meyers, V., & Elfferich, I. (2001). Near-death experience in survivors of cardiac arrest: A prospective study in the Netherlands. *Lancet, 358,* 2039–2045, Parnia, S., & Fenwick, P. (2002). Near death experiences in cardiac arrest: Visions of a dying brain or visions of a new science of consciousness. *Resuscitation, 52*(1), 5–11.

8. Sabom, M. (1982). *Recollections of death: A medical investigation.* New York, NY: Simon & Schuster.

9. Sartori, P. (2008). The near-death experiences of hospitalized intensive care patients: A five-year clinical study. Lewiston, NY: Edwin Mellen Press.

10. Holden, J. M. (2009). Veridical perception in near-death experiences. In J. M. Holden, B. Greyson, & D. James (Eds.), *The handbook of near-death experiences: Thirty years of investigation.* Santa Barbara, CA: Praeger/ABC-CLIO:185–211.

11. Long, J., & Perry, P. (2010). *Evidence of the afterlife: The science of near-death experiences.* New York, NY: HarperCollins: 74–78.

12. Van Lommel, P., van Wees, R., Meyers, V., & Elfferich, I. (2001). Near-death experience in survivors of cardiac arrest: A prospective study in the Netherlands. *Lancet, 358,* 2039–2045.

13. Cook, E. W., Greyson, B., & Stevenson, I. (1998). Do any near-death experiences provide evidence for the survival of human personality after death? Relevant features and illustrative case reports. *Journal of Scientific Exploration,12,* 377–406; and Kelly, E. W., Greyson, B., & Stevenson, I. (1999–2000). Can experiences near death furnish evidence of life after death? *Omega, 40*(4), 513–519.

14. Cook, E. W., Greyson, B., & Stevenson, I. (1998). Do any near-death experiences provide evidence for the survival of human personality after death? Relevant features and illustrative case reports. *Journal of Scientific Exploration, 12,* 399–400.

15. Ring K., & Cooper S. (1999). *Mindsight: Near-death and out-of-body experiences in the blind.* Palo Alto, CA: William James Center for Consciousness Studies.

16. Paraphrased. Full text of original account is at: www.nderf.org/NDERF/NDE_Experiences/marta_g_nde.htm.

17. John, E. R., Prichep, L. S., Kox, W., Valdes-Sosa, P., Bosch-Bayard, J., Aubert, E., Tom, M., diMichele, F., & Gugino, L. D. (2001). Invariant reversible QEEG effects of anesthetics. *Consciousness & Cognition, 10,* 165–183.

18. White, N. S., & Alkire, M. T. (2003). Impaired thalamocortical connectivity in humans during general-anesthetic-induced unconsciousness. *NeuroImage, 19,* 402–411.

19. Long, J., & Perry, P. (2010). *Evidence of the afterlife: The science of near-death experiences.* New York, NY: HarperCollins: 98.

20. Greyson, B., Kelly, E. W., & Kelly, E. F. (2009). Explanatory models for near-death experiences. In J. M. Holden, B. Greyson, & D. James (Eds.), *The handbook of near-death experiences: Thirty years of investigation.* Santa Barbara, CA: Praeger/ABC-CLIO: 226.

21. Long, J., & Perry, P. (2010). *Evidence of the afterlife: The science of near-death experiences.* New York, NY: HarperCollins: 111.

22. Long, J., & Perry, P. (2010). *Evidence of the afterlife: The science of near-death experiences.* New York, NY: HarperCollins: 125.

23. Kelly, E. W. (2001). Near-death experiences with reports of meeting deceased people. *Death Studies, 25,* 229–249.

24. Long, J., & Perry, P. (2010). *Evidence of the afterlife: The science of near-death experiences.* New York, NY: HarperCollins:123–124.

25. Osis, K., & Haraldsson, E. (1977). *At the hour of death* (3rd ed.). New York, NY: Avon.

26. Greyson, B. (2010). Seeing deceased persons not known to have died: "Peak in Darien" experiences. *Anthropology & Humanism, 35,* 159–171.

27. Long, J., & Perry, P. (2010). *Evidence of the afterlife: The science of near-death experiences.* New York, NY: HarperCollins:137–139.

28. Sutherland, C. (2009). *Trailing clouds of glory: The near-death experiences of Western children and teens.* In J. M. Holden, B. Greyson, & D. James (Eds.), *The handbook of near-death experiences: Thirty years of investigation.* Santa Barbara, CA: Praeger/ABC-CLIO: 93.

29. Long, J, & Perry, P. (2010). *Evidence of the afterlife: The science of near-death experiences.* New York, NY: HarperCollins: 151–159.

30. Holden, J., Long, J., & MacLurg, J. (2009). Characteristics of Western near-death experiencers. In J. M. Holden, B. Greyson, & D. James (Eds.), *The handbook of near-death experiences: Thirty years of investigation.* Santa Barbara, CA: Praeger/ABC-CLIO: 110.

31. Long, J., & Perry, P. (2010). *Evidence of the afterlife: The science of near-death experiences.* New York, NY: HarperCollins: 166. The NDERF website has a compilation of non-Western NDEs shared with NDERF at: http://www.nderf.org/NDERF/Research/non_western_ndes.htm.

32. Fracasso, C., Aleyasin, S., Friedman, H., & Young, M. (2010). Near-death experiences among a sample of Iranian Muslims. *Journal of Near-Death Studies, 29,* 271.

33. Nahm, M., & Nicolay, J. (2010). Essential features of eight published Muslim near-death experiences: An addendum to Joel Ibrahim Kreps's "The search for Muslim near-death experiences." *Journal of Near-Death Studies, 29,* 255.

Chapter Eight: Apparently Non-Physical Veridical Perception in Near-Death Experiences

The author wishes to thank J. Kenneth Arnette, Robert Mays, Suzanne Mays, and Titus Rivas for their helpful comments in the preparation of this chapter.

1. Moody, R. A., Jr. (1975). *Life after life.* Covington, GA: Mockingbird Books.

2. Holden, J. M. (2009). Veridical perception in near-death experiences. In J. M. Holden, B. Greyson, & D. James (Eds.), *The handbook of near-death experiences: Thirty years of investigation.* Santa Barbara, CA: Praeger/ABC-CLIO: 185–211.

3. Sartori, P. (2004). A prospective study of NDEs in an intensive therapy unit. *Christian Parapsychologist, 16,* 34–40.

4. Zingrone, N. L., & Alvarado, C. S. (2009). Pleasurable Western adult near-death experiences: Features, circumstances, and incidence. In J. M. Holden, B. Greyson, & D. James (Eds.), *The handbook of near-death experiences: Thirty years of investigation.* Santa Barbara, CA: Praeger/ABC-CLIO: 17–40.

5. Sabom, M. (1982). *Recollections of death: A medical investigation.* New York, NY: Simon & Schuster.

6. Wiltse, A. S. (1889). A case of typhoid fever, with subnormal temperature and pulse. *The St. Louis Medical and Surgical Journal, 57,* 281–288, 355–64.

7. Myers, F. W. H. (1892). On indications of continued Terrene knowledge on the part of the phantasms of the dead. *Proceedings of the Society for Psychical Research, 8,* 170–252.

8. Barkallah, S. (Producer/Director). (2015). *Untimely departure* [Motion picture, English translation]. Berre l'Etang, France: S17. Retrieved from http://www.nderf.org/NDERF/NDE_Experiences/departed_sonia. htm

9. Neal, M. (2012). *To heaven and back: A doctor's extraordinary account of her death, heaven, angels, and life again: A true story.* Multnomah, OR: WaterBrook Press.

10. Greyson, B. (2010). Seeing dead people not known to have died: "Peak in Darien" experiences. *Anthropology and Humanism,* 35, 159–171. doi: 10.1111/j.1548-1409.2010.01064.x

11. Burpo, T., & Vincent, L. (2010). *Heaven is for real.* Nashville, TN: Thomas Nelson.

12. Rush, M. J. (2013). Critique of "A prospectively studied near-death experience with corroborated out-of-body perceptions and unexplained healing." *Journal of Near-Death Studies, 32,* 3–14.

13. Rush, M. J. (2013). *Rejoinder to "Response to 'Critique of "A* prospectively studied near-death experience with corroborated out-of-body perceptions and unexplained healing."'" *Journal of Near-Death Studies, 32, 37–41.*

14. Sartori, P. (2013). Response to "Critique of 'A prospectively studied near-death experience with corroborated out-of-body perceptions and unexplained healing.'" *Journal of Near-Death Studies, 32,* 15–36.

15. Smit, R. H. (2008). Corroboration of the dentures anecdote involving veridical perception in an NDE. *Journal of Near-Death Studies, 27,* 47–61.

16. Smit, R. H., & Rivas T. (2010). Rejoinder to "Response to 'Corroboration of the dentures anecdote involving veridical perception in a near-death experience.'" *Journal of Near-Death Studies, 28,* 193–205.

17. Woerlee, G. M. (2010). Response to "Corroboration of the dentures anecdote involving veridical perception in a near-death experience." *Journal of Near-Death Studies, 28,* 181–191.

18. Holden, J. M. (1988). Visual perception during naturalistic near-death out-of-body experiences. *Journal of Near-Death Studies,* 7, 107–120. doi:10.1007/BF01073945

19. Holden, J. M., & Joesten, L. (1990). Near-death veridicality research in the hospital setting: Problems and promise. *Journal of Near-Death Studies, 9,* 45–54. doi: 10.1007/BF01074101

20. Lawrence, M. (1996, August). *Prospective NDE studies with AIDS and cardiac patients.* Paper presented at the International Association for Near-Death Studies North American Conference, Oakland, CA.

21. Lawrence, M. (1997). *In a world of their own: Experiencing unconsciousness.* Westport, CT: Praeger.

22. Parnia, S., Waller, D. G., Yeates, R., & Fenwick, P. (2001). A qualitative and quantitative study of the incidence, features and aetiology of near death experiences in cardiac arrest survivors. *Resuscitation,* 48, 149–156.

23. Parnia, S., & Fenwick, P. (2002). Near death experiences in cardiac arrest: Visions of a dying brain or visions of a new science of consciousness. *Resuscitation, 52,* 5–11.

24. Sartori, P., Badham, P., & Fenwick, P. (2006). A prospectively studied near-death experience with corroborated out-of-body perceptions and unexplained healing. *Journal of Near-Death Studies, 25,* 69–84.

25. Greyson, B., Holden, J. M., & Mounsey, J. P. (2006). Failure to elicit near-death experiences in induced cardiac arrest. *Journal of Near-Death Studies, 25,* 85–98.

26. Parnia, S., Spearpoint, K., de Vos, G., Fenwick, P., Goldberg, D., Yang, J., et al, & Schoenfeld, E. R. (2014). AWARE—AWAreness during Resuscitation—A prospective study. *Resuscitation,* 85, 1790–1805.

27. Greyson, B. (1983). The near-death experience scale: Construction, reliability, and validity. *Journal of Nervous and Mental Disease, 171,* 369–375.

28. Lange, R., Greyson, B., & Houran, J. (2004). A Rasch scaling validation of a "core" near-death experience. *British Journal of Psychology, 95,* 161–177.

29. Van Lommel, P., van Wees, R., Meyers, V., & Elfferich, I. (2001). Near-death experience in survivors of cardiac arrest: A prospective study in the Netherlands. *Lancet, 358,* 2039–2045.

30. Rivas, T., Dirven, A., & Smit, R. *What a dying brain can't do: Evidence of paranormal phenomena involving near-death experiences* (W. Boeke, Trans.). Manuscript in preparation.

31. Holden, J. M, Hupfeld, K., Lawson, E., Mays, R., Mays, S., Rivas, T., & Kinsey, L. *Apparently non-physical veridical perception during near-death experiences: An analysis of cases from the professional literature.* Manuscript in preparation.

Chapter Nine: Through the Eyes of a Child: Near-Death Experiences in the Young

1. Moody, R. A., Jr. (1975). *Life after life.* Covington, GA: Mockingbird Books; Ring, K. (1980). *Life at death: A scientific investigation of the near-death experience.* New York, NY: Coward, McCann and Geoghegan; Sabom, M. (1982). *Recollections of death:*

An investigation revealing striking new medical evidence of life after death. London, UK: Corgi. (First publication in Great Britain); Morse, M., & Perry, P. (2000). *Where God lives: The science of the paranormal and how our brains are linked to the universe.* New York, NY: Cliff Street Books. (An imprint of HarperCollins Publishers)

2. Van Lommel, P., van Wees, R., Meyers, V., & Eifferich, I. (2001, December 15). Near-death experience in survivors of cardiac arrest: A prospective study in the Netherlands. *The Lancet, 358*, 2039–2045; Parnia, S., Waller, D. G., Yeates, R., & Fenwick, P. (2001). A qualitative and quantitative study of the incidence, features and aetiology of near death experiences in cardiac arrest survivors. *Resuscitation, 48*, 149–156; Parnia, S., Spearpoint, K., de Vos, G., Fenwick, P., et al. (2014). AWARE—AWAreness during Resuscitation—A prospective study. *Resuscitation* (in press accepted 7 September 2014); Schwaninger, J., Eisenberg, P. R., Schechtman, K. B., & Weiss, A. N. (2002, Summer). A prospective analysis of near-death experiences in cardiac arrest patients. *Journal of Near-Death Studies, 20*(4), 215–232; Greyson, B. (2003). Incidence and correlates of near-death experiences in a cardiac care unit. *General Hospital Psychiatry, 25*, 269–276; Sartori, P. (2008). *The near-death experiences of hospitalized intensive care patients: A five-year clinical study.* New York, NY/Lampeter, Wales, UK: The Edwin Mellen Press.

3. Herzog, D., & Herrin, J. (1985). Near-death experiences in the very young. *Critical Care Medicine, 13*(12), 1074–1075; Ring, K. & Valarino, E. (1998). *Lessons from the light.* New York, NY/London, UK: Insight Books, Plenum Press: 108–112; Serdahely, W. J. (1995). Variations from the prototypic near-death experience: The "individually tailored" hypothesis. *Journal of Near-Death Studies, 13*, 185–96; Sutherland, C. (1995). *Children of the light: The near-death experiences of children.* Sydney, Australia: Bantam Books.

4. Morse, M., Conner, D., & Tyler, D. (1985). Near-death experiences in a pediatric population. *American Journal of Diseases of Children, 139*, 595–600; Morse, M., Castillo, P., Venecia, D., Milstein, J., & Tyler, D. C. (1986). Childhood near-death experiences. *American Journal of Diseases of Children, 140*, 1110–1114. Morse, M., & Perry, P. (1990). *Closer to the light: Learning from children's near-death experiences.* New York, NY: Villard Books.

5. Sutherland, C. (1992). *Transformed by the light: Life after near-death experiences.* Sydney, Australia: Bantam Books. (U.S. ed. pub. [1995b] *Reborn in the light: Life after near-death experiences.* New York, NY; Toronto, Canada; London, UK; Sydney, Australia; Auckland, New Zealand: Bantam Books); Sutherland, C. (1995a). *Children of the light: The near-death experiences of children.* Sydney, Australia: Bantam Books.

6. Atwater, P. M. H. (1995). A call to reconsider the field of near-death studies. *Journal of Near-Death Studies, 14*, 5–15; Atwater, P. M. H. (1999). *Children of the new millennium: Children's near-death experiences and the evolution of humankind.* New York, NY: Three Rivers Press.

7. Bush, N. E. (1983). The near death experience in children: Shades of the prison-house reopening. *Anabiosis: The Journal of Near Death Studies, 3*, 177–193.

8. Serdahely, W. J. (1989–1990). A pediatric near-death experience: Tunnel variants. *Omega, 20*(1), 55–62; Serdahely, W. J. (1990). Pediatric near-death experiences. *Journal of Near-Death Studies, 9*(1), 33–39.

9. Gabbard, G. O., & Twemlow, S. W. (1984). *With the eyes of the mind: An empirical analysis of out-of-body states.* New York: Praeger.

10. Burpo, T., & Vincent, L. (2010). *Heaven is for real.* Nashville, TN: Thomas Nelson.

11. Sartori, P. (2014). *The wisdom of near-death experiences: How understanding NDEs can help us live more fully.* London, UK: Watkins Publishing: 58.

12. Burpo, T., & Vincent, L. (2010). *Heaven is for real.* Nashville, TN: Thomas Nelson; Malarkey, K., & Malarkey, A. (2010). *The boy who came back from heaven: A remarkable account of miracles, angels, and life beyond this world.* Carol Stream, IL: Tyndale House Publishers.

13. Burpo, T., & Vincent, L. (2010). *Heaven is for real.* Nashville, TN: Thomas Nelson.

14. Atwater, P. M. H. (1995). A call to reconsider the field of near-death studies. *Journal of Near-Death Studies, 14,* 10; Bush, N. E. (1983). The near death experience in children: Shades of the prison-house reopening. *Anabiosis: The Journal of Near Death Studies, 3,* 177–193; Morse, M., Castillo, P., Venecia, D., Milstein, J., & Tyler, D. C. (1986). Childhood near-death experiences. *American Journal of Diseases of Children, 140,* 1110–1114.

15. Sutherland, C. (1995a). *Children of the light: The near-death experiences of children.* Sydney, Australia: Bantam Books: 99–100; Morse, M. with Perry, P. (1992). *Transformed by the light.* London: Piatkus.

16. Atwater, P. M. H. (1999). *Children of the new millennium: Children's near-death experiences and the evolution of humankind.* New York, NY: Three Rivers Press: 42.

17. Bush, N. E. (1983). The near death experience in children: Shades of the prison-house reopening. *Anabiosis: The Journal of Near Death Studies, 3,* 177–193; Morse, M. (1994). Near death experiences and death related visions: Implications for the clinician. *Current Problems in Pediatrics.* Feb 1994, pp. 55–83; Serdahely, W.J. (1991) A Comparison of retrospective accounts of childhood near-death experiences with contemporary pediatric near-death experience accounts. *Journal of Near-Death Studies, 9*(4), pp. 219-224.

18. Greyson, B., & Bush, N. E. (1992). Distressing near-death experiences. *Psychiatry: Interpersonal and Biological Processes, 55*(1), 95–110.

19. Morse, M., Conner, D., & Tyler, D. (1985). Near-death experiences in a pediatric population. *American Journal of Diseases of Children, 139,* 595–600; Morse, M., Castillo, P., Venecia, D., Milstein, J., & Tyler, D. C. (1986). Childhood near-death experiences. *American Journal of Diseases of Children, 140,* 1110–1114; Morse, M., & Perry, P. (1990). *Closer to the light: Learning from children's near-death experiences.* New York, NY: Villard Books.

20. Morse, M., & Perry, P. (1990). *Closer to the light: Learning from children's near-death experiences.* New York, NY: Villard Books.

21. Morse, M., & Perry, P. (2000). *Where God lives: The science of the paranormal and how our brains are linked to the universe.* New York, NY: Cliff Street Books. (An imprint of HarperCollins Publishers)

22. Atwater, P. M. H. (1999). *Children of the new millennium: Children's near-death experiences and the evolution of humankind.* New York, NY: Three Rivers Press: 93.

23. Sutherland, C. (1992). *Transformed by the light: Life after near-death experiences.* Sydney, Australia: Bantam Books. (U.S. ed. pub. [1995b] *Reborn in the light: Life after near-death experiences.* New York, NY; Toronto, Canada; London, UK; Sydney, Australia; Auckland, New Zealand: Bantam Books); Sutherland, C. (1995a). *Children of the light: The near-death experiences of children.* Sydney, Australia: Bantam Books.

Chapter Ten: Distressing Near-Death Experiences: The Basics

Originally published November/December 2014, *Missouri Medicine*, 111, 6.

1. Greyson B., & Bush, N. E. (1992). Distressing near-death experiences. *Psychiatry*, 55, 95–110.

2. Bush, N. (2012). *Dancing past the dark: Distressing near-death experiences.* Cleveland, TN: Parson's Porch Books.

3. Storm, H. (2001). *My descent into death: A second chance at life.* East Sussex, UK: Clairview.

4. Rommer, B. (2001). *Blessings in disguise: Another side of the near-death experience.* St. Paul, MN: Llewellyn.

5. Sharp, K. C. (1986). In C. F. Flynn, *After the Beyond: Human transformation and the near-death experience.* Englewood Cliffs, NJ: Prentice-Hall, p. 85.

6. Corbett, L. (1996). *The religious function of the psyche.* London, UK: Routledge.

7. Ingall, M. (2000, July). Stairway to heaven. *Mademoiselle*, 94–86.

8. Joseph, S. (2013). *What doesn't kill us: The new psychology of posttraumatic growth.* New York, NY: Basic Books.

9. Wren-Lewis, J. (2004). The implications of near-death experiences for understanding posttraumatic growth. *Psychological Inquiry*, *15*, 90–92.

10. Bush, N. E. (2009). *Distressing Western near-death experiences: Finding a way through the abyss.* In J. M. Holden, B. Greyson, & D. James (Eds.), *The handbook of near-death experiences: Thirty years of investigation.* Santa Barbara, CA: Praeger/ABC-CLIO: 63–96.

11. Cressy, J. (1994). *The near-death experience: Mysticism or madness.* Hanover, MA: Christopher Publishing House.

12. Flynn, C. P. (1986). *After the beyond: Human transformation and the near-death experience.* Englewood Cliffs, NJ: Prentice-Hall.

13. Moody, R. A., Jr. (2013). Near-death experiences: An essay in medicine and philosophy. *Missouri Medicine*, *110*, 368–371.

Chapter Eleven: Near-Death Experiences: The Mind-Body Debate & the Nature of Reality

Originally published July/August 2015, *Missouri Medicine*; Vol. 114: 4.

1. Alexander, E. (2012). *Proof of heaven: A neurosurgeon's journey into the afterlife.* New York, NY: Simon & Schuster.

2. Alexander, Eben, III. (2012). My Experience in Coma. *AANS Neurosurgeon, 21*(2).

3. Carter, Chris. (2012). *Science and the afterlife experience: Evidence for the immortality of consciousness.* Rochester, VT: Inner Traditions.

4. Holden, J. M., Greyson, B., & James, D. (Eds). (2009). *The handbook of near-death experiences: Thirty years of investigation.* Santa Barbara, CA: Praeger/ABC-CLIO.

5. Moody, R. A., Jr. (2001). *Life after life: The investigation of a phenomenon—survival of bodily death.* New York, NY: HarperCollins Publishers. (Originally published in 1975 by MBB, Inc., and later by Bantam Books, a division of Bantam Doubleday Dell Publishing Group, Inc., in 1976)

6. Moody, R. A., Jr., & Perry, P. (2010). *Glimpses of eternity: Sharing a loved one's passage from this life to the next.* New York, NY: Guideposts.

7. Tucker, J. B. (2013). *Return to life: Extraordinary cases of children who remember past lives.* New York, NY: St Martin's Press.

8. Van Lommel, P. (2010). *Consciousness beyond life: The science of the near-death experience* (L. Vroomen, Trans.). New York, NY: HarperCollins. (Originally published as *Eindeloos bewustzijn: Een wetenschappelijke visie op de bijna-dood ervaring* in 2007 by Kampen, The Netherlands: Ten Have Publishing)

9. Chalmers, D. J. (1996). *The conscious mind: In search of a fundamental theory.* Oxford, UK: Oxford University Press.

10. Baker, M. C., & Goetz, S. (2011). *The soul hypothesis: Investigations into the existence of the soul.* London, UK: The Continuum International Publishing Group.

11. Cardeña, E., et al. (2014, January). A call for an open, informed study of all aspects of consciousness. *Frontiers in Human Neuroscience, 8*(17), 1–4.

12. Jahn, R. G., & Dunne, B. J. (1987). *Margins of reality: The role of consciousness in the physical world.* New York, NY: Harcourt, Brace, Jovanovich.

13. Kelly, E. F., Kelly, E. W., Crabtree, A., Gauld, A., Grosso, M., & Greyson, B. (Eds.). (2007). *Irreducible mind: Toward a psychology for the 21st century.* Lanham, MD: Rowman & Littlefield.

14. Kelly, E. F., Crabtree, A., & Marshall, P. (Eds.). (2014). *Beyond physicalism: Toward reconciliation of science and spirituality.* Lanham, MD: Rowman & Littlefield.

15. Penrose, R., Longair, M., Shimony, A., Cartwright, N., & Hawking, S. (1997). *The large, the small, and the human mind.* Cambridge, UK: Cambridge University Press.

16. Penfield, W. (1975). *The mystery of the mind: A critical study of consciousness and the human brain.* Princeton, NJ: Princeton University Press, 1975.

17. Lockwood, M. (1989). *Mind, brain & the quantum: The compound "I."* Oxford, UK: Basil Blackwell, Ltd.

18. Sheehan, D. P. (Proceedings editor). (2006). *Frontiers of time: Retrocausation—experiment and theory, University of San Diego, San Diego, California, 20–22 June 2006. AIP Conference Proceedings, 863.*

19. Sheehan, D. P. (Proceedings editor). (2011). *Quantum retrocausation—Theory and experiment, American Institute of Physics, University of San Diego, San Diego, California, 13–14 June 2011.* ISBN: 978-0-7354-0981-1. *AIP Conference Proceedings* for 92nd Meeting of AAAS Pacific Division.

20. Rosenblum, B., & Kuttner, F. (2006). *Quantum enigma: Physics encounters consciousness.* New York, NY: Oxford University Press.

Chapter Twelve: Neuroscience Perspectives on Near-Death Experiences
Originally published March/April 2015, *Missouri Medicine, 112*, 2.

1. James, W. (1902). *The varieties of religious experience.* Longmans, Green, and Co.

2. Owens, J. E., Cook, E. W., & Stevenson I. (1990). Features of "near-death experience" in relation to whether or not patients were near death. *Lancet*, 336, 1175–1177.

3. Dostoyevsky, F. (1959). *The idiot* (C. Garnett, Trans.). New York: Dell.

4. Frank, J. (1983). *Dostoevsky: The years of ordeal, 1850–1859.* Princeton, NJ: Princeton University Press.

5. Van Lommel, P., van Wees, R., Meyers, V., & Elfferich, I. (2001). Near-death experience in survivors of cardiac arrest: A prospective study in the Netherlands. *Lancet, 358*, 2039–2045.

6. Parnia, S., Waller, D. G., Yeates, R., & Fenwick, P. (2001). A qualitative and quantitative study of the incidence, features and aetiology of near death experiences in cardiac arrest survivors. *Resuscitation, 48*, 149–156.

7. Greyson, B. (2003). Incidence and correlates of near-death experiences in a cardiac care unit. *General Hospital Psychiatry, 25*, 269–276.

8. Nelson, K. R., Mattingly, M., Lee, S. A., & Schmitt F. A. (2006). Does the arousal system contribute to near-death experience? *Neurology, 66*, 1003–1009.

9. Lempert, T., Bauer, M., & Schmidt, D. (1994). Syncope and near-death experience. *Lancet, 344*, 829–830.

10. Lempert, T., Bauer, M., & Schmidt, D. (1994). Syncope: A videometric analysis of 56 episodes of transient cerebral hypoxia. *Annals of Neurology, 36*, 233–237.

11. Ohayon, M. M. (2000). Prevalence of hallucinations and their pathological associations in the general population. *Psychiatry Research, 97*, 153–164.

12. Nelson, K. R., Mattingly, M., Schmitt, F. A. (2007). Out-of-body experience and arousal. *Neurology, 68*, 794–795.

13. Descartes, R. (1996). *Meditations on first philosophy with selections from the objections and replies* (J. Cottingham, Ed. and Trans.) (Rev. ed., with introduction by B. A. O. Williams). New York, NY: Cambridge University Press.

14. Blanke, O., Ortigue, S., Landis, T., & Seeck, M. (2002). Stimulating illusory own-body perceptions. *Nature*, 419, 269–270.

15. Blanke, O., Landis, T., Spinelli, L., & Seeck, M. (2004). Out-of-body experience and autoscopy of neurological origin. *Brain, 127*, 243–258.

16. Stace, W. T. (1960). *Mysticism and philosophy.* London: Macmillan.

17. Hood, R. W., Ghorbani, N., Watson, P. J., et al. (2001). Dimensions of the mysticism scale: Confirming the three-factor structure in the United States and Iran. *Journal for the Scientific Study of Religion, 40*, 691–705.

18. Lempert, T., & von Brevern, M. (1996). The eye movements of syncope. *Neurology, 46*, 1086–1088.

19. Moody, R. A., Jr. (1975). *Life after life.* Covington, GA: Mockingbird Books.

20. Kroeger, D., Florea, B., & Amzica, F. (2013). Human brain activity patterns beyond the isoelectric line of extreme deep coma. *PLoS ONE, 8*, e75257.

21. Van Lommel, P. (2010). *Consciousness beyond life: The science of the near-death experience* (L. Vroomen, Trans.). New York, NY: HarperCollins. (Originally published as *Eindeloos bewustzijn: Een wetenschappelijke visie op de bijna-dood ervaring* in 2007 by Kampen, The Netherlands: Ten Have Publishing)

22. Alexander, E. (2012). *Proof of heaven: A neurosurgeon's journey into the afterlife.* New York, NY: Simon & Schuster.

23. Sacks, O. W. (2012, December 12) Seeing God in the third millennium: How the brain creates out of body experiences and religious epiphanies. *The Atlantic.*

24. Penfield, W. (1975). *The mystery of the mind: A critical study of consciousness and the human brain.* Princeton, NJ: Princeton University Press.

25. Kandel, E. R. (1998). A new intellectual framework for psychiatry. *American Journal of Psychiatry, 155*, 457–469.

26. Gottlieb, R. (2014, November 6). Back from heaven: The science. *The New York Review of Books.*

27. Nelson, K. R. (2011). *The spiritual doorway in the brain: A neurologist's search for the God experience.* New York, NY: Penguin Group.

28. Nelson, K. R. (2014). Near-death experience: arising from the borderlands of consciousness in crisis. *Annals of the New York Academy of Sciences, 1330*, 111–119.

29. Mahowald, M. W., & Schenck, C. H. (1992). Dissociated states of wakefulness and sleep. *Neurology, 42*, 44–51.

30. Overeem, S., Mignot, E., van Dijk, J. G., & Lammers, G. J. (2001). Narcolepsy: Clinical features, new pathophysiologic insights, and future perspectives. *Journal of Clinical Neurophysiology, 18*, 78–105.

31. LaBerge, S., Levitan, L., Brylowski, A., & Dement, W. (1988). "Out-of-body" experiences occurring in REM sleep. *Sleep Research*, 17, 115.

32. Cheyne, J. A., & Girard, T. A. (2009). The body unbound: Vestibular-motor hallucinations and out-of-body experiences. *Cortex, 45*, 201–215.

33. Maquet, P., Ruby, P., Maudoux, A., et al. (2005). Human cognition during REM sleep and the activity profile within frontal and parietal cortices: A reappraisal of functional neuroimaging data. *Progress in Brain Research, 150*, 219–227.

Chapter Thirteen: Near-Death Experiences and the Emerging Scientific View of Consciousness

Originally published July/August 2015, *Missouri Medicine, 112*, 4.

I wish to thank Bruce Greyson, MD, Edward F. Kelly, PhD, and Neal Grossman, PhD, for their thoughtful comments that aided in the preparation of this manuscript.

1. Chalmers, D. J. (1996). The conscious mind: In search of a fundamental theory. Oxford, UK: Oxford University Press.

2. Merrill, P. W. (1940). *Spectra of long-period variable stars.* Chicago, IL: University of Chicago Press.

3. Kelly, E. F., Kelly, E. W., Crabtree, A., Gauld, A., Grosso, M., & Greyson, B. (2007). *Irreducible mind: Toward a psychology for the 21st century.* Lanham, MD: Rowman & Littlefield.

4. Holden, J. M., Greyson, B., & James, D. (Eds). (2009). *The handbook of near-death experiences: Thirty years of investigation.* Santa Barbara, CA: Praeger/ABC-CLIO.

5. Owens, J. E., Cook, E. W., & Stevenson, I. (1990). Features of "near-death experience" in relation to whether or not patients were near death. *Lancet, 336*: 1175–1177.

6. Greyson, B., & Long, J. P. (2006). Does the arousal system contribute to the near-death experience? *Neurology, 66*: 2265

7. Alexander, E. (2012). *Proof of heaven: A neurosurgeon's journey into the afterlife.* New York, NY: Simon & Schuster.

8. Penfield, W. (1975). *The mystery of the mind: A critical study of consciousness and the human brain.* Princeton, NJ: Princeton University Press.

9. Koch, C. (2012). *Consciousness: Confessions of a romantic reductionist.* Cambridge, MA: Massachusetts Institute of Technology Press.

10. Rosenblum, B., & Kuttner, F. (2006). *Quantum enigma: Physics encounters consciousness.* New York, NY: Oxford University Press.

11. Ringbauer, M., Duffus B., Branciard C., Cavalcanti E. G., White A. G., & Fedrizzi, A. (2015, January 20). Measurements on the reality of the wavefunction, *Natural Physics*, 11, 249–254.

12. Sheehan, D. P. (Proceedings editor). (2006). *Frontiers of time: Retrocausation—experiment and theory, University of San Diego, San Diego, California, 20–22 June 2006. AIP Conference Proceedings, 863.*

13. Sheehan, D. P. (Proceedings editor). (2011). *Quantum retrocausation—Theory and experiment, American Institute of Physics, University of San Diego, San Diego, California, 13–14 June 2011.* ISBN: 978-0-7354-0981-1. *AIP Conference Proceedings* for 92nd Meeting of AAAS Pacific Division.

14. Moody, R. A., Jr., & Perry, P. (2010). *Glimpses of eternity: Sharing a loved one's passage from this life to the next.* New York, NY: Guideposts.

15. Gottlieb, R. (2014, November 6). Back from heaven: The science. *The New York Review of Books.*

16. Dossey, L. (2013). *One mind: How our individual mind is part of a greater consciousness and why it matters.* Carlsbad, CA: Hay House, Inc.

17. Kelly, E. F., Crabtree, A., & Marshall, P. (Eds.). (2014). *Beyond physicalism: Toward reconciliation of science and spirituality.* Lanham, MD: Rowman & Littlefield.

18. Cardeña, E., et al. (2014, January). A call for an open, informed study of all aspects of consciousness. *Frontiers in Human Neuroscience*, 8(17), 1–4.

Index

Note: Page numbers in italics refer to figures or tables.

Index

Index

Index